REPLACEMENT THERAPY

Sixth Edition

by   Puthygraman K. Natrajan, M.D.
Associate Clinical Professor
Department of Obstetrics and Gynecology
& Physiology and Endocrinology
1980 – 2003
Medical College of Georgia
Augusta, GA 30912-3396

and   R. Don Gambrell, Jr., M.D.
Clinical Professor
Department of Obstetrics and Gynecology
& Physiology and Endocrinology
1978 – 2001
Medical College of Georgia
Augusta, GA 30912-3396

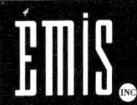 medical publishers

For Direct Mail Orders, write:

**EMIS, Inc.
Medical Publishers**
P.O. Box 820062
Dallas, TX 75382-0062

Telephone Orders
1 800 225 0694

FAX Orders
214 349 2266

Online Orders
www.emispub.com

ISBN: 0-917634-34-9

SIXTH EDITION

Copyright R. DON GAMBRELL, JR., M.D., and PUTHY-GRAMAN K. NATRAJAN, M.D., Augusta, GA, 2005. All rights reserved. No part of this publication may be reproduced, stored in a retrieval system or transmitted in any form or by any means, electronic, mechanical, photocopying, recording or otherwise, without the prior written permission of the publisher.

TRADEMARKS: All brand and product names are trademarks or registered trademarks of their respective companies. It has been attempted throughout this text to distinguish proprietary trademarks from generic and/or descriptive terms by following the capitalization style used by the manufacturer; however, EMIS, Inc. cannot attest to the accuracy of this information. Use of a term in this text should not be regarded as affecting the validity of any trademark or service mark.

Printed on recycled paper
Published in the United States 2005

DEDICATION

This book is dedicated to our wives, *Caroline Gambrell*, who for more than 40 years has supported my every endeavor with love, warmth, and kind understanding.

∼

Bhuvana Natrajan, who has been a great support for more than 23 years.

∼

It is also dedicated to *Dr. Robert B. Greenblatt,* our mentor, who is the Father of Reproductive Endocrinology and Hormone Replacement Therapy in the United States.

TABLE OF CONTENTS

Dedication iii

Indications
   Introduction 2
   Vasomotor Symptoms 6
   Urogenital Atrophy 8
   Psychogenic Manifestations 10
   Osteoporosis 14
   Coronary Artery Disease (CAD) 20
   Alzheimer's Disease (AD) 26
   The Women's Health Initiative (WHI) 30

Evaluation
   Vaginal Hormonal Cytology 46
   Progestogen Challenge Test 48
   Endometrial Biopsy 52
   Osteoporosis Detection Methods 56
   Laboratory and Tests for Early
      Cancer Detection 62

Hormone Replacement
   Oral Estrogens 66
   Non-Oral Estrogens 70
   Androgens 78
   Progestogens 86
   Selective Estrogen Receptor Modulators (SERMS) . 92
   Oral Contraceptives 94

Calcium
   Calcium Supplements 96

Risks
   Endometrial Hyperplasia 100
   Endometrial Cancer 104
   Hormones and Breast Cancer 112
   Thromboembolic Disease 122
   Hypertension 124
   Gallbladder Disease 126
   Nutrition and Diet 128
   Lipid Metabolism 130

Side Effects
   Management of Side Effects 134

Contraindications.......................... 138
Alternative Therapy 142
References
References................................ 146
Listing of Manufacturers..................... 166

TABLES

TABLE 5.1: Approved Recommendations:
   National Osteoporosis Foundation............... 19
TABLE 5.2: Approved Therapeutic Options
   For Osteoporosis 19
TABLE 5.3: Treatment Reduction: Fractures 19
TABLE 6.1: Nurses Health Study: Mortality 24
TABLE 14.1: Oral Estrogens 68
TABLE 14.2: Estrogen - Progestogen................ 69
TABLE 15.1: Estrogen Vaginal Creams and Rings 74
TABLE 15.2: Parenteral Intramuscular Estrogens.......75
TABLE 15.3: Transdermal Estrogens 76
TABLE 15.4: Transdermal Estrogen-Progestogen 77
TABLE 16.1: Androgens........................... 82
TABLE 17.1: Progestogens......................... 91
TABLE 20.1: Calcium Supplements.................. 99
TABLE 21.1: Effects of Progestogens on
   Endometrial Hyperplasia..................... 102
TABLE 21.2: Reversal of Hyperplasia
   with Increased Duration of Progestogens 103
TABLE 22.1: Incidence of Endometrial
   Cancer at Wilford Hall USAF Medical Center 108
TABLE 23.1: Incidence of Breast Cancer at
   Wilford Hall USAF Medical Center 118

FIGURES

FIGURE 1.1: Age of Menopause 5
FIGURE 7.1: ET/HT Use and AD Risk 28
FIGURE 8.1: Cumulative Number of Breast
   Cancers Diagnosed in 1000 Women 40

FIGURE 8.2: Risk Estimates: Mortality/
   Survival: Estrogen + Progestin 41
FIGURE 8.3: Risk Estimates: Breast Cancer-
   Unopposed Estrogens 42
FIGURE 8.4: Risk Estimates: Breast Cancer-
   Estrogen + Progestin 43
FIGURE 8.5: Secondary Prevention of
   CVD Mortality............................. 44
FIGURE 22.1: Incidence of Endometrial Cancer....... 109
FIGURE 22.2: Changing Incidence of
   Endometrial Cancer......................... 110
FIGURE 23.1: Incidence of Cancer:Age 119
FIGURE 23.2: Incidence of Breast Cancer
   Treatment Group 120
FIGURE 23.3: Incidence of Breast Cancer: Estrogen
   and Estrogen-Progestogen Treated............... 121
FIGURE 28.1: Changes in Lipoproteins............. 131

EMIS, Inc. Books 168

SECTION 1: INTRODUCTION

Menopausal Hormone Deficiency

On average women cease to menstruate by age 51.2 years. The symptoms of 'menopause' may start as early as age 40 in some women. Many of them will spend one-third of their life after menopause. However, women's experience of the menopause and its effects on their remaining years vary widely (see Figure 1.1).

The declining ovarian function can be rapid for some and slower for others. Some women may produce sufficient endogenous estrogens to remain asymptomatic, but others develop a variety of disturbances during the *climacteric*, a term in current use for the pre-menopausal, menopausal, and postmenopausal period.

These symptoms may include:
- Hot flushes (or flashes)
- Night sweats
- Vaginal irritation or dryness
- Insomnia
- Depression
- Fatigue
- Urinary symptoms
- Palpitations
- Anxiety
- Irritability
- Mood swings
- Headache

The issue of what should be done about adverse climacteric symptoms is controversial. There is general agreement that menopause is a hormone-deficient state and should be treated. Physicians are now asking what dosages of estrogen should be used and what regimens of hormone replacement are best for their patients.

It is no longer contended that menopausal symptoms are psychoneurotic. It is no longer thought that only vasomotor manifestations (hot flushes, sweats) and atrophic vaginitis are directly due to the estrogen deficit, and that these manifestations may be treated with a smallest possible dose of oral estrogens, and/or vaginal estrogens, for a short period of time.

Trends in Treatment

Estrogen replacement therapy is controversial. It was fashionable in the 1960s, but in the 1970s complications became apparent. Physicians became reluctant to treat the climacteric, and patients became wary of hormone therapy because of widely publicized reports that estrogens cause endometrial cancer. In the 1980s, however, hormone therapy grew in popularity, and this trend continued until recently. The publications of the The Heart and Estrogen/Progestin Replacement Study (HERS) and Women's Health Initiative (WHI) studies have raised some doubt about the increased risk of hormone therapy, but estrogen therapy continues to be popular among many patients.

First, there has been a growing recognition of the dangers of long-term estrogen deficiency, which can lead to development of:

- Osteoporosis and related fracture complications
- Atherosclerotic heart disease
- Psychogenic manifestations
- Alzheimer's disease

Although it has not been directly shown that estrogen deficiency increases the risk for colon cancer, several new studies have observed that therapy with any sex steroid (estrogen, progestogen, or androgen) decreases the risk for colon cancer (see Section 12).

There is growing acknowledgment that estrogen deficiency should be treated as vigorously as any other endocrinopathy and without a limitation of time. Instead of the minimal treatments suggested in the past to alleviate specific symptoms, some women require hormonal therapy:

- For years instead of months
- Continuously instead of cyclically
- In larger dosages than were previously recommended

Further, there is a recognition that some postmenopausal women need treatment with other hormones (e.g., progestogen) to prevent endometrial hyperplasia and subsequent neoplasia.

Second, the belief that estrogen treatment causes endometrial cancer is no longer valid. The incidence of cancer of the endometrium, or of the breast, need not increase as a result of long-term estrogen therapy if cyclic progestogens in adequate dosages are added to the estrogen regimen.

FIGURE 1.1—Age Of Menopause

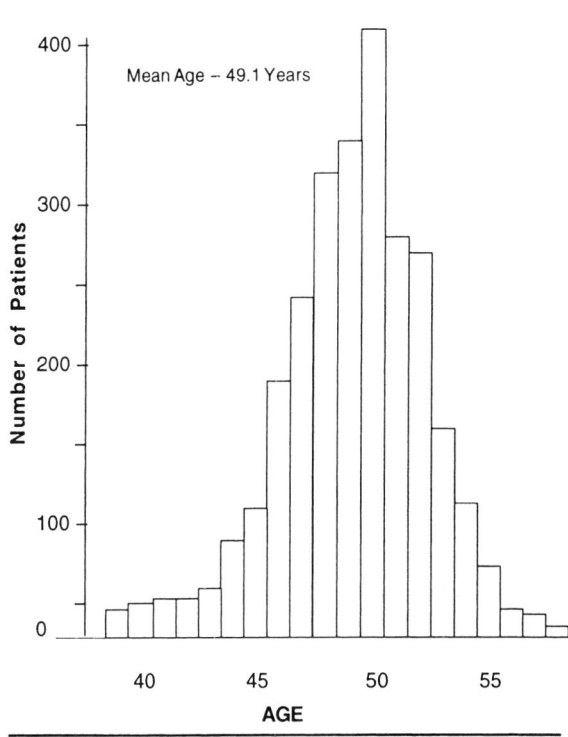

The age of menopause in more than 2,000 women undergoing natural menopause. (Reproduced with permission of the publisher; The American Fertility Society, from Gambrell) {45}

SECTION 2: VASOMOTOR SYMPTOMS

Clinical Information

Most women who seek medical attention for menopausal symptoms complain of vasomotor symptoms. These include:
- Hot flushes (or flashes)
- Night sweats

These symptoms usually:
- Have an insidious onset
- Increase as serum estrogens decline
- Are variable in frequency and severity
- May persist for several months to a few years

Research

Other studies have shown an association between the pulsatile release of LH and the occurrence of hot flushes. However, LH levels in and of themselves are not responsible for triggering vasomotor symptoms, since these phenomena can occur after hypophysectomy. Some studies have shown that the hot flashes are due to lack of catechol estrogens. In the brain estrogens are converted to catechol estrogens. The catechol estrogens prevent the conversion of tyrosine to norepinephrine or adrenaline. When there is an estrogen deficiency there is increased levels of norepinephrine and this may lead to hot flashes. If untreated, the hypothalamus and autonomic nervous systems gradually adjust to the lower levels of estrogen and eventually hot flushes abate.

Patients with gonadal dysgenesis have high levels of gonadotropins. However, these individuals experience vasomotor symptoms only after exposure to exogenous estrogens and subsequent withdrawal.

Recommendations

In the past, low dosages of estrogen have been given for short intervals and then reduced gradually so that hot flushes fade. This concept is no longer valid. A woman experiencing menopausal symptoms has become estrogen-deficient and will remain so for the rest of her life.

A balanced program of estrogen replacement therapy combined with cyclic progestogens is the best treatment, since the real goal of estrogen replacement is not only to alleviate vasomotor symptoms, but to prevent later metabolic consequences, such as osteoporosis and atherosclerosis.

SECTION 3: UROGENITAL ATROPHY

Clinical Information
Atrophy of the genital epithelium may result in senile vaginitis. Symptoms may include:
- Irritation
- Burning
- Pruritus
- Leukorrhea
- Dyspareunia
- Vaginal bleeding
- Decrease of vaginal secretions
- Thinning and easily-traumatized epithelium
- Shortening and lessening of distensibility of the vagina

Most sexual problems experienced by postmenopausal women are due to the physical status of the vaginal mucosa, which must maintain sufficient protective moisture and provide lubrication during coitus. After menopause, atrophic changes may lead to:
- Dyspareunia
- Vaginitis
- Vaginismus
- Physical discomfort
- Loss of sexual interest

Research
Studies have demonstrated {134} that the estrogen-deprived state in postmenopausal women leads to changes in:
- Quantity of vaginal fluid
- pH levels
- Vaginal blood flow

However, urogenital changes that develop because of estrogen deprivation are reversible with estrogen replacement therapy, although the longer the estrogen deprivation, the slower the physiologic response.

Recommendations

The preferred treatment for atrophic vaginitis is local estrogen therapy in the form of vaginal creams (e.g., *Premarin* and *Estrace*), which are well absorbed into the vaginal mucosa. Daily bedtime applications should be given for one to two weeks, thereafter applications three times per week are normally sufficient for maintenance. There are estradiol vaginal tablets available to use twice a week, *Vagifem*, or an estradiol ring to be inserted and removed every three months—*Estring* or *Femring*—(see Section 14).

Systemic therapy by oral or other routes is usually started simultaneously. Local vaginal therapy can sometimes be discontinued after a few months, or continued vaginal cream treatment may be required in addition to systemic estrogens. Irritative symptoms abate rapidly with estrogen vaginal cream, but restoration of normal vaginal blood flow may take up to a year.

To a lesser extent, the vulvar epithelium also becomes thin and may be irritated or subject to infection. These conditions commonly respond to applications of vaginal estrogen cream, but a one- or two-percent testosterone cream may be necessary for kraurosis vulva or other atrophic or leukoplakic vulvar conditions. Vulvar pruritus may sometimes require one-percent hydrocortisone creams or other glucocorticoid creams for relief in addition to either estrogen or testosterone creams.

The integrity of the lower urinary tract mucosa is dependent upon estrogens. Estrogen deficiency may therefore result in irritative symptoms such as:

- Dysuria
- Burning on urination
- Cystitis
- Urethral caruncles
- Nongonococcal urethritis

These symptoms respond best to local applications of vaginal estrogens in different forms, with the simultaneous initiation of oral estrogen therapy.

SECTION 4: PSYCHOGENIC MANIFESTATIONS

Clinical Information

Many postmenopausal women complain of psychogenic disturbances. These may include:
- Increased nervousness
- Depression
- Anxiety
- Insomnia
- Headaches
- Mood swings

In one study the tryptophan and free tryptophan was decreased in estrogen deprived patients; once estrogen therapy was begun these levels increased alleviating depression in many patients {58}. Other conditions that may be aggravated by menopausal symptoms include:
- Pre-existing psychosomatic problems intensified by hot flushes
- Sleep patterns disturbed by night sweats
- Decreased libido due to atrophic vaginitis and dyspareunia

Research

Carefully controlled double-blind and crossover studies indicate that estrogens have a tonic mental effect {33}. Estrogen patients had higher scores on psychometric evaluations, alleviating the psychogenic manifestations independent of vasomotor symptoms {15}

Moderate to severe depression, as measured by the Zung Self-Rating Depression Scale, was significantly higher in patients who had surgical menopause by hysterectomy with or without bilateral oophorectomy compared to women undergoing natural menopause {3}. This suggests that women undergoing pelvic surgery have either not been reconciled to its necessity or were insufficiently prepared for its consequences.

In a study using pellets of estradiol, testosterone, or placebo, testosterone increased the frequency and intensity of orgasmic responses {153}. In a double-blind study using hot flushes as the main index, 96 percent of patients improved on estrogens and 91 percent on an estrogen-androgen combination. Fair to good results were obtained in 56 percent of patients receiving androgens, and 16 percent of those were given a placebo. The estrogen-androgen combination was associated with less withdrawal bleeding, and accentuated well-being and healthy libido {154}.

Headaches in postmenopausal women are frequently regarded as psychosomatic and not hormone-related; but in one study using estrogen, progestogen, and placebo, headaches were alleviated while high levels of estrogen were maintained {33}.

In a study of 85 patients receiving hormone replacement therapy when headaches were a secondary complaint, relief from headaches was obtained by the administration of estradiol pellets alone or in combination with testosterone {58}.

Although these studies may not prove that psychogenic complaints of postmenopausal women are hormone-dependent, they indicate that many are hormone-responsive, since patients improve once therapy is begun.

Recommendations

Sexual dysfunction in menopausal women, long regarded by psychologists and sex therapists as psychogenic, has been shown to be responsive to hormone therapy. Relief may be afforded by:
- Estrogens, including estrogen vaginal cream, for complaints such as:
  - Vaginal dryness
  - Dyspareunia
- Androgens, for complaints of loss of sexual interest (see Section 16)
- Use of local testosterone cream, *Sildenafil Vaginal Cream,* or enhancement cream compounded by a pharmacist can add to sexual response. *Avlimil* is

a tablet that is available through the internet site www.Avlimil.com.

It is important to note that a postmenopausal woman who has lost up to two-thirds of estrogen production has also lost up to one-half of androgen production. Although most postmenopausal women respond well to estrogen-progestogen therapy, some require the addition of an androgen. Women treated with estrogen-androgen replacement therapy were more composed, elated, and energetic than those treated with estrogen alone {142}. The addition of androgen enhanced sexual desire and increased the frequency of sexual fantasies compared to estrogen alone, or with placebo. In the *Yale Mid-Life Study Program*, androgens are not routinely prescribed unless there is a deficiency in the total or free testosterone levels {134}.

NOTES

SECTION 5: OSTEOPOROSIS

Introduction

Osteoporosis is a silent disease which affects over ten million Americans. Seventy-five percent of them are women. Unfortunately in many, the earliest sign is a debilitating fracture of hip or spine. There are over ten million women with osteoporosis and 34 million with low bone mass (osteopenia), which leads to osteoporosis. Many of these women can be treated early to prevent the devastating fractures. There are 1.5 million women who will develop osteoporotive fractures compared to 300,000 women with heart disease and 180,000 breast cancers. It is estimated that 50% of women age 50 and over will develop a fracture during their life time.

What is Osteoporosis?

With osteoporosis there is a reduction in the quantity of bone and a deterioration of not only the main structure, but also the micro architecture of bone tissue. This causes fragility of bone and increases the risk of fractures. It affects up to ten million postmenopausal Caucasian women. Women of Asian descent also have a high risk of developing osteoporosis {91}. There are approximately 1.5 million fractures ascribed to osteoporosis, of which 300,000 are hip fractures, and about twenty-five percent of patients die in one year. About one out of every six Caucasian women will develop a hip fracture. Only about fifteen percent will return to a normal life style.

Vertebral fractures cause major physical disabilities like:
- severe back pain
- height loss
- posture change (Dowager's Hump)

Also, breathing problems due to compression of the chest, and secondary to fractures and abdominal problems are due to fracture in the lumbar region. All of these can reduce the quality of life.

Risk Factors

Women reach their peak bone mass around thirty years of age. Genetic predisposition, poor nutrition, (especially lack of calcium intake), lack of exercise, exposure to alcohol and smoking, all affect the bone mass. After loss of estrogen during menopause all women lose bone for the first three to five years at an accelerated rate, and after that at a slower rate throughout their life. Other factors, such as thyroid excess, arthritis, bowel disease, etc., cause increased bone loss.

Diagnosis

The current gold standard is measurement of bone density with DEXA scan of spine and hip but other modalities like peripheral scans with DEXA or ultrasound can also be used. There are other bone density measurements which can be used, such as peripheral single or dual energy x-ray absorptiometry, computerized tomography (QCT) and ultrasound. The National Osteoporosis Foundation recommends that all women get a bone density test after age 65, regardless of other risk factors. Women under age 65, with one or more additional risk factors, need a bone density test.

Peripheral techniques include measurement in forearm, tibia, wrist, finger or heel. Markers of bone turnover in urine or serum are sometimes used to help assess the fracture risk, predict bone loss or assess response to treatment, but they do not replace bone density testing.

The goal of management in osteoporosis is prevention.

Reduction of Risk Factors

Recommendations to reduce the risk of osteoporosis include:

- Discontinue smoking
- Reduce risk of falls in the home by ensuring there is adequate lighting and clear passages
- Daily calcium intake = 1000–1500 mg
- Daily Vitamin D intake = 400 IU
- Adequate nutrition, e.g., milk, fruits and vegetables

- Daily weight bearing exercise, such as walking, golf, tennis, etc.
- Eliminate alcohol

When to Treat

We treat osteoporosis in women who have:
- experienced fractures,
- have a bone density T-Score of less than, or equal to, 2.5 standard deviations (SD),
- have a T-Score of less than, or equal to, 1.5 SD with additional risk factors.

Approved Medications

Approved medications for prevention, treatment and reduction of hip and spine fractures include:
- *Estrogen* — oral and transdermal
- *Raloxifen* — oral
- *Calcitonin* — nasal spray
- *Alendronate* — oral
- *Risedronate* — oral
- *Ibandronate* — oral
- *Terapeptide* — injection (Parathyroid Hormone)

Estrogens:

A metanalysis by Torgerson and Bell-Syer examined 22 studies and revealed that non-vertebral factures were reduced by 27 percent in *estrogen* treated women compared to controls {163}.

Results from the WHI trial indicated that hormone replacement therapy reduced the risk of hip fracture by 34 percent and all fractures by 24 percent {131}.

SERMS:

The Selective Estrogen Receptor Modulators (SERMS) have some estrogenic effect. *Raloxifen* is currently approved for prevention and treatment of osteoporosis. The Multiple Outcome of Raloxifen Evaluation (MORE) trial showed that *Raloxifen* produced modest effects on bone density and reduced bone turnover marker. *Raloxifen* reduces vertebral fracture, but has not been shown to reduce hip fractures.

Calcitonin:

Calcitonin inhibits osteoclast function, thus reduces bone loss. It is available in injectable or nasal spray form. In the Prevent Recurrence of Osteoporosis Fractures (PROOF) study nasal calcitonin decreases vertebral fractures, but it has not been shown to decrease the hip fractures effectively; it is an option in women who cannot tolerate other modalities.

Biphosphonates:

These are compounds which inhibit bone resorption.

Alendronate:

Alendronate is a potent inhibitor. In the Fracture Intervention Trial (FIT) women increased bone density significantly: 7 to 9% per year at spine, and 5–8% per year in hip, compared to placebo. It has also been shown to reduce the risk of hip fractures by 56% without prior vertebral factures. New vertebral factures were reduced by 50% {9}. Metanalysis of several clinical trials showed consistent reduction of hip fractures by 50% and significant reduction in vertebral and wrist fractures.

Discontinuation of *alendronate* does not result in accelerated loss of bone seen in women who discontinue estrogen {162}. It can be used in a daily dose of 10 mg or 70 mg once a week. It should be taken with water, on an empty stomach, in the morning; no other food or drink should be taken for thirty minutes. To prevent irritation of the esophagus the patient should not lie down.

Risedronate:

Risedronate is an equally effective bisphonate compound that is used in a dose of 5 mg per day, or 35 mg once-a-week. The Vertebral Efficacy with Resideronate Threrapy

(VERT) trial indicates vertebral fractures were reduced by 40% at three years. In the hip intervention program there was a reduction of hip fractures by 40%.

Recombinent Parathormone (PTH):
Parathyroid hormone regulates calcium homeostasis and is the only available bone stimulating agent. It not only increases bone mass, but also seems to restore bone architecture. In the Recombinent Parathormone (PTH) study, women who had previous fractures, vertebral fractures, were reduced by 60 to 65% and non-vertebral fractures were reduced by 35 to 45%.

Conclusion
Osteoporosis is a debilitating disease. The best way to avoid complications is by prevention by reducing risk factors and addition of medications, as necessary, at an early stage.

TABLE 5.1: APPROVED RECOMMENDATIONS OF NATIONAL OSTEOPOROSIS FOUNDATION

1. Discuss risk of osteoporosis
2. Record height and discuss skeletal health
3. Patients with fractures: measure BMD
4. Recommend BMD for all women over 65
5. Recommend BMD for women below 65 with risk factors
6. Advise calcium intake 1200 mg per day
7. Regular weight bearing exercise
8. Avoid tobacco and alcohol
9. Suggest therapy—with BMD "T" Score less than 2.0 and BMD less than 1.5 with risk factors

TABLE 5.2: APPROVED THERAPEUTIC OPTIONS FOR OSTEOPOROSIS

	Prevention	**Treatment**
Estrogen	Yes	No
Raloxifene	Yes	Yes
Calcitonin (Nasal Spray)	No	Yes
Alendronate	Yes	Yes
Risedronate	Yes	Yes
Terapeptide	No	Yes

TABLE 5.3: TREATMENT REDUCTION OF FRACTURES

Approved Option	**Hip**	**Spine**
Estrogens	No	No
Raloxifene	No	Yes
Calcitonin (Nasal Spray)	No	No
Alendronate	Yes	Yes
Risdronate	No	Yes
Terapeptide	No	Yes

SECTION 6: CORONARY ARTERY DISEASE (CAD)

Clinical Information

The greatest benefit that will accrue to postmenopausal estrogen users is prevention of coronary artery disease (CAD), in spite of current controversies. More than 100 studies of all types—clinical, epidemiologic, angiographic, basic sciences, animal experimentation, and laboratory—indicate at least a 50 percent reduction in heart disease and stroke. Myocardial infarction rarely occurs in young women prior to menopause. Younger women who have had bilateral oophorectomy demonstrate a higher incidence of myocardial infarction unless estrogen therapy is begun soon after the ovaries are removed. More than 450,000 women die every year in the U.S. from heart disease and stroke; many of these deaths are preventable.

There have been several recent studies that have shown detrimental effects of continuous combined HRT therapy on heart disease and stroke, but not with unopposed estrogen. The HERS I Study was a secondary prevention trial in postmenopausal women who had a cardiac event (mean age 67 years). The initial study ended after 4.1 years of follow-up. There was an increase in cardiac events during the first year, but a reduced risk after years three and four. The study was continued as HERS II for 2.7 years, but there was a high drop-out rate after the first year—from 81% to 45%. In both HERS I and HERS II there was a non-significant increased risk of CAD, and a non-significant increased risk of stroke.

In the WHI study there was increased risk of CAD and stroke. This would result in seven more cardiac events and eleven more strokes per 10,000 women each year, compared to placebo. At the study entry 7.7% had prior cardiovascular disease (CVD), and were older with a mean age of 63.3 years. The 29% increase in heart disease was in those who used continuous combined estrogen/progestogen therapy, but not the *Premarin* users.

There were fewer deaths from CVD in HRT users compared to those given placebo. These findings led the WHI investigators, as well as others, to recommend against hormone therapy for primary prevention of heart disease or stroke.

Prevention

Several studies suggest that estrogens may exert a protective effect against CVD and stroke, especially when low dosages of natural estrogens sufficient to relieve menopausal symptoms are used. In a review of epidemiologic evidence, although most studies observed significant protection, cross-sectional and prospective external control studies observed the lowest relative risks from 0.3 to 0.4 {146}. Perhaps the best studies are provided by the cohort studies with internal controls (RR = 0.58; 95 percent CI, 0.48 – 0.70). A summary estimate of all studies omitting the hospital-based case control studies yielded an RR of 0.52.

The Nurses' Health Study {147} confirmed that:
- Ever estrogen use significantly reduced the risk of coronary artery disease (RR = 0.5; P = 0.007)
- Current estrogen use reduced the risk even lower (RR = 0.3; P = 0.001)
- These benefits held after adjustments for factors such as:
  - Smoking
  - Hypertension
  - Diabetes
  - High cholesterol
  - Parental history of myocardial infarction
  - Previous use of oral contraceptives
  - Obesity

In addition to prevention of CVD, all causes of mortality were reduced significantly; 37 percent in the estrogen users of the Nurses' Health Study, with more than 20 years of follow-up (see Table 6.1). With long-term use of more than ten years, mortality was reduced by 20 percent. Death from heart disease was reduced by 49 percent; and although not quite statistically significant, death from stroke was reduced in the estrogen users by 32 percent. Even cancer mortality (endometrial, breast, ovarian and colorectal cancers) was significantly reduced by 29 percent. Although breast cancer deaths decreased by 24 percent, at this point in their follow-up, this was not statistically significant.

Angiography Studies

At least three cardiology studies using angiography have observed less coronary artery occlusion in estrogen users (61, 100, 156}. A 56- to 63 percent reduction in risk for developing severe coronary artery stenosis in women who used estrogen was observed. Sullivan et al assessed the 10-year survival rate of 2,268 menopausal women who had varying degrees of angiographically defined coronary artery atherosclerosis with respect to estrogen use. In women without demonstrable CAD at the initial angiogram, there was no statistically significant difference in the 10-year survival rate of never-users (85 percent, n = 347) vs ever-users (95.6 percent, n = 99). However, in women with more than 70-percent lumen stenosis at the initial angiogram, the 10-year survival rate of never-users dropped to 60 percent (n = 1,108) and was significantly less than the 97-percent, 10-year survival rate among ever users (n = 70; P = 0.027) (see Figure 8.5). In another study, the age-adjusted odds ratios for use of postmenopausal estrogen among women with moderate and severe levels of occlusion of coronary arteries were 0.59 (95% CI, 0.48 to 0.73) and 0.37 (95% CI, 0.29 to 0.46), respectively, which indicated a statistically significant protective effect of postmenopausal estrogen on coronary occlusion.

Animal Experimentation

Animal studies using cynomolgus macaque monkeys fed an atherogenic diet found that male and ovariectomized female monkeys did not differ with respect to coronary artery atherosclerosis, while premenopausal females had half the CAD of their counterparts. Hormone replacement therapy halved the extent of coronary artery atherosclerosis in oophorectomized monkeys compared to control animals.

In delineating some of the mechanisms of coronary vessel protection, acetylcholine produced vasoconstriction of coronary arteries in postmenopausal monkeys; but when estrogen was replaced, there was coronary vasodilation. When medroxyprogesterone acetate was added to estrogen replacement therapy, there was neither vasodilation nor vasoconstriction to acetylcholine. However, there was some suggestion that monkeys treated with conjugated estrogens and medroxyprogesterone acetate had larger lumens than monkeys treated with estrogen alone.

Estrogen use also reduces the risk of cerebrovascular disease, but this has not been observed in every study. In the study that used the general population as a comparison group, there was a significantly decreased risk of stroke (RR = 0.54; 95% CI, 0.24 to 0.84). In the four prospective studies using internal controls, all found estrogen use to be beneficial, with RRs ranging from 0.23 to 0.63 {68,69,116,117}. Both the Nurses' Health Study and the Framingham Study failed to find decreased risk of stroke in estrogen users {147, 173}. In the Leisure World Study, protection from stroke was observed in all age groups except the youngest (RR = 0.53; 95 percent CI, 0.31 to 0.91) {114}. This decreased risk was unaltered by adjustments for possible confounding variables such as:
- Smoking
- Alcohol
- Body mass
- Exercise

Direct Effects of Estrogen

Although from 25 to 50 percent of the effect of estrogen on CVD is mediated through improved lipid patterns, there are also direct effects, such as:
- Estrogen and progesterone receptors identified in coronary vessel walls
- Improved vascular blood flow
- Dilation of coronary arteries
- Increased EDRF (endothelial-derived relaxing factor)
- Reduced vascular resistance

- Increased velocity of blood flow
- Increased cardiac output
- Inhibited atherosclerosis progression
- Decreased platelet adhesiveness
- Inhibited coronary thrombosis
- Prostacyclin and thromboxane metabolism
- Peripheral vasodilation

TABLE 6.1: NURSES' HEALTH STUDY MORTALITY DATA {62}

Cause Of Death	RR	95% CI
All Cause Mortality in Current Hormone Users	0.63	0.56–0.70
Long-term Use More Than 10 Years	0.80	0.67–0.96
Heart Disease in Current Users	0.51	0.45–0.57
Stroke in Current Users	0.68	0.39–1.16
All Cancers in Current Users	0.71	0.62–0.81
Breast Cancer in Current Users	0.76	0.56–1.02

NOTES

SECTION 7: ALZHEIMER'S DISEASE (AD)

Clinical Information

There is considerable evidence that estrogen has an effect on the central nervous system (CNS). Estrogen deficiency may contribute to the neurodegenerative changes of the aging CNS and increase the incidence of senile dementia of the Alzheimer's type. The incidence of Alzheimer's Disease (AD) increases more in women than in men after age 65, so that age-specific rates vary from 1.5 to 3.0 times that of men.

Research

Two of the many findings in AD are a decrease in dendritic spines and a deficiency of the cholinesterase enzymes necessary to reconvert the neurotransmitters to acetyl choline. Studies in oophorectomized animals indicate that axonal and/or dendritic growth of cholinergic neurons and acetyl cholinesterase processes increased in the estrogen-treated animals, while in controls, the acetyl cholinesterase reaction was essentially localized only on cell bodies {73}. These cholinergic nuclei in the brain are involved in most memory functions, and this population of cells undergoes the most pronounced degenerative changes seen in AD.

Some but not all clinical studies have observed that estrogen therapy improves cognitive function. In a study of 65-year-old women, estrogen users had significantly higher scores on short- and long-term verbal memory tasks compared to women who had never used estrogen {82}. However, no differences were found between estrogen users and non-users on measures of visual/spatial memory.

In a Japanese study of seven women with AD, six showed improvement in dementia ($P \leq 0.05$) {72}. In a study of women with dementia, none of the 158 cases were currently using estrogen, whereas 15 percent of the matched controls were {8}. The resulting relative risk of dementia in women taking estrogens was RR = 0.07 ($P \leq 0.001$).

The Leisure World studies observed a 30-percent reduction of AD in estrogen users {113}. In a study of 2,529 female cohort members who died, the risk of AD and related dementia was less in estrogen users compared to non-users (RR = 0.69; 95% CI, 0.46 to 1.03). The risk decreased significantly with increasing estrogen dosage and duration of use.

A large prospective study of 1,124 elderly women indicated that the age of onset of AD was significantly later in women who had taken estrogen than in those who had not (RR = 0.4; 95% CI, 0.22 to 0.85) {157}.

Another epidemiologic study did not observe any reduction in AD with estrogen use {140}.

In a study of 107 female AD cases, the RR was 1.1 (95 percent CI, 0.6 to 1.8). However, this study only evaluated ever estrogen use, including vaginal estrogen cream, while the Leisure World study observed the greatest decrease with increasing estrogen dosage and duration of use.

Recently the WHI studies have shown a slightly increased risk of "probable" dementia in women (average age 72 years) taking estrogen. RR–2.05; 95% CI, 1.21–3.48. They estimated that there would be 23 additional cases of AD per 10,000 women per year. Regarding AD, it is very important at which age estrogen therapy is initiated. The Cache County study had previously shown that if estrogen replacement was not initiated until after age 60, AD was increased 112% {177}. Although none of the women in The Women's Health Initiative Memory Study (WHIMS) had overt Alzheimer's at the beginning of the trial, all were age 65 or older, and had never used estrogen, so the change to the brain had already occurred. They missed the window of opportunity to impact their lifetime risk of AD by 83 percent. The probable impact of this report is that there will be millions more cases of AD because of this report.

There is increasing evidence from large epidemiologic studies that estrogen may exert protective effects on the human brain. For example, the use of HRT and ERT in healthy postmenopausal women may reduce:

- The prevalence of AD
- The risk of developing AD
- Delay the onset of AD {69}

A longitudinal PET (Positron Emission Tomography) study lasting two years was done to examine the effect of estrogen replacement on regional cerebral blood flow during memory tasks {96}. Regional cerebral blood flow in the hippocampus, para hippocampal gyrus and temporal lobes was significantly higher in users of HRT compared with non-users. Another group conducted a longitudinal observational study to investigate the effect of long-term HRT in glucose metabolism in three brain regions, previously reported to decline with advancing age. After two years, the HRT users (both estrogen and combined therapy) had a significantly increased rate of glucose metabolism in the lateral temporal region, whereas non-users and males did not {163}.

FIGURE 7.1—ET/HT Use and AD Risk

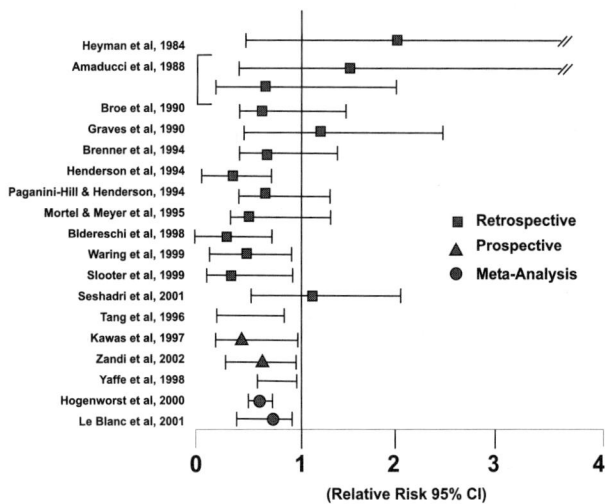

NOTES

SECTION 8: THE WOMEN'S HEALTH INITIATIVE (WHI) REPORTS IN PERSPECTIVE

Facts or Fallacies?

R. Don Gambrell Jr. M.D.

Women's concern about hormone use increased following early termination of the estrogen/progestogen arm of the Women's Health Initiative (WHI) {131}. Prior to the report of the WHI in July 2002, it was estimated that 15 million postmenopausal women were using estrogens because multiple studies and decades of use had demonstrated a balance of benefits and risks. With the wide media coverage it was estimated that up to 50 percent of the 15 million women using hormones stopped. Many women stopped therapy without even discussing it with their physician. Furthermore, so many doctors were so uncertain about how to respond, some even advised their patients to discontinue their hormones. The report of the WHI investigators was pre-empted by a press conference that prejudges the meaning of the data for our patients and us {152}. Media reports glossed over the benefits for bone mass, decrease in colon cancer, and fewer deaths among the users vs the controls, to emphasize the risks for breast cancer and cardiovascular disease. It was a classical case of symbolism over substance, where hype fomented hysteria.

On March 2, 2004, the National Institutes of Health (NIH) announced that it was stopping the estrogen-only, *Premarin,* phase of the of the WHI because estrogen alone does not affect the risk of heart disease or breast cancer {159}. After nearly seven years, the outcomes indicated:

Coronary Heart Disease (CHD)	HR = 0.91; 95% CI, 0.75–1.12
Breast Cancer	HR = 0.77; 95% CI, 0.59–1.01
Stroke (121 more strokes per 10,000 women per year)	HR = 1.39; 95% CI, 1.10–1.77
Hip Fractures	HR = 0.61; 95% CI, 0.41–0.91
Dementia	HR = 1.49; 95% CI, 0.83–2.66

What is the Women's Health Initiative, and why do many adverse reports continue to be released from the National Heart, Lung and Blood Institute? The WHI was designed more than ten years ago, 1992, as a primary prevention trial with a planned duration of 8.5 years, comparing estrogen use alone, *Premarin*, or combined estrogen-progestogen therapy, *PremPro*, to placebo. Expected outcomes included development of heart disease, breast cancer, stroke, blood clots, endometrial cancer, colorectal cancer and deaths due to other cancers.

A Data Safety Monitoring Board (DSMB) set statistical risk levels for the two primary end points, breast cancer and CVD. The DSMB set safety thresholds that were very conservative so that if one of these critical values was observed, the committee was obligated to stop the study. The breast cancer hazard ratio (HR), or relative risk of 1.26, with 95% CI of 1.00–1.59, exceeded the Board's predetermined threshold; hence the study was halted. It should be pointed out the HR was not statistically significant since the 95% CI included 1.00. When the other risk factors for breast cancer were added, the results lost even borderline significance because the 95% CI decreased to 0.83–1.92. The press conference and the report stated that the trial was stopped early because the health risks exceeded the health benefits. Unfortunately, most patients, and many physicians, believed that the trial was stopped because it showed that hormones caused breast cancer. However, this was not new data. The collaborative group on hormonal factors in breast cancer reported in 1997 an increased risk after five years of estrogen use. (RR = 1.115; 95% CI, 1.011–1.80). (See Figure 8.1); {25}. The report also listed the other HRs:

Coronary Heart Disease (CHD):	1.29; 95% CI, 1.02–1.63
Stroke:	1.41; 95% CI, 1.07–1.85
Pulmonary Embolism:	2.13; 95% CI, 1.39–3.25

However, these ratios did not trigger the predetermined safety threshold that would have halted the study. Even so, they have become whips in the stampede to proclaim hormone replacement unsafe. All that can really be said is, "at the end of the 5.2-year average observation period, the statistical analysis for these occurrences suggested harm". Because the study was never completed, i.e., the duration upon which the initial hypotheses were built was not fulfilled, the primary outcome measure, a benefit or lack of benefit from estrogen plus progestin, MHT for nonfatal myocardial infarction and coronary heart disease (CHD) was neither proven or disproved.{152}

Death Rates

Total mortality was decreased in the *PremPro* users to a HR = 0.98; 95% CI, 0.82–1.18. In the women with breast cancer there were three deaths in the hormone users and two deaths in the controls. A previous report in 2001 by a respected epidemiologist observed a lower risk of death from breast cancer in hormone users when compared to nonusers (Figure 8.2) {12}. This study also evaluated all 55 of the prior studies of breast cancer in estrogen users and found no increased risk. (Figures 8.3, 8.4). The WHI was too short in duration (5.2 years with some women taking PremPro only 2–3 years) to determine much of anything about breast cancer. When a cancer in the breast can be diagnosed by palpation, that tumor has been developing for seven to eight years based on doubling times. Mammograms will detect cancers two to three years earlier, which is why annual mammograms are so important. There are now more than 60 published studies indicating that estrogen can be safely given to women with previous breast cancer {88}. In this review, there were 21 studies with sufficient data for comparison: 152 of the 1,612 estrogen users with previous breast cancer had recurrences (9.4%), while 739 of the 3,640 controls had either recurrence or new breast cancers (20.3%).

The 29 percent increase in heart disease, or seven more events per 10,000 women per year, is probably true since this has been shown in the HERS study {77}, and is also biologically explainable, whereas breast cancer is not. Although estrogens have beneficial effects in cardiovascular diseases by increasing HDL cholesterol and decreasing LDL cholesterol, the major benefit is through direct effects of estrogen upon the coronary arteries. Most hormones work through receptors in target tissues. Estrogen increases its receptors in coronary arteries where progestogens decrease the estrogen receptors, particularly when taken continuously as they are with *PremPro*. This may leave fewer sites for the estrogen beneficial action; increased blood flow, dilation of coronary arteries, reduced vascular resistance, increased velocity of blood flow, inhibition of atherosclerosis progression, decreased platelet adhesiveness, and increased peripheral vasodilation.

WHI findings do not apply to most users of hormone therapy. Because of the characteristics of the WHI study population, results cannot be compared to the typical hormone therapy users, i.e., the woman who is seeking relief from menopausal symptoms. Women with significant menopausal symptoms, especially hot flashes, were excluded from the WHI. In addition, the average age of women in the WHI was 63 years, so many already had increased risk for heart disease, such as progressive atherosclerosis, with some even having prior angioplasty or coronary bypass surgery. Studies in younger postmenopausal women, with an average age of 53 years, although using *PremPro,* or other estrogen-progestogen regimens, do not find any increase in heart disease. It should be emphasized that in the WHI, the study in the *Premarin only* users was not stopped in July 2002 because they did not have any increase in either breast cancer or heart disease. They were to be continued on estrogen alone for at least another 3 years, but were stopped in March 2004 because after seven years of use, and with an average age of 70, there was no increased risk for heart disease or breast cancer. {159}

Even with the alleged findings of increased breast cancer and heart disease, there were several benefits in the WHI, where absolute risk reductions per 10,000 patients were six fewer colorectal cancers, 5 fewer hip fractures, and fewer deaths in the *PremPro* users, compared to non-users. While up to 50 percent of the 15 million estrogen users stopped their hormones after the WHI report, some have resumed therapy. It is now estimated that seven-to-eight-million women in the United States are taking estrogens. Many who had stopped their therapy are again using estrogens because of unbearable symptoms. In a recent report it was estimated that where there were 91 million new HRT prescriptions in 2001, only 57 million new HRT prescriptions were written in 2003; a 42% decrease {70}. Of this decrease 80% were for *Premarin* or *PremPro*. Transdermal and vaginal estrogen prescriptions remained steady because of a slight increase in vaginal estrogen use; however, these only account for 10% of all new HRT prescriptions. The WHI was thought to be such a well-designed study that it would answer the remaining questions about estrogen use. With its many flaws, the WHI has raised more questions than answers. The information gleaned from multiple studies of so many different hormones and methods of administration for the past 50 years should not be discounted because of a single study. Although large, only two different hormones and one method of administration was used, i.e., continuous oral administration. It should be emphasized that the DMSB did not find any adverse events during 5.2 years of *Premarin* use, so these women were continued on that estrogen for a total of seven years, until March 2004.

The report of the Women's Health Initiative Memory Study (WHIMS) in May 2003 may have the most devastating impact on postmenopausal health of all the WHI reports {139}. Contrary to multiple previous studies of estrogen therapy and AD, the WHI observed a 105 percent increase in AD. The age estrogen is started is most important. If estrogen therapy is started at menopause, there is an 83 percent reduction in the lifetime risk of AD, but when started after age 60 this may not occur because the changes in the brain have already begun {177}. In the WHIMS all the women were age 65 or older when estrogen was initiated. They did not have overt AD, but the changes in the brain had already occurred. In the *Premarin only* WHIMS study there was also an increase in dementia, but it was only a HR of 1.49; 95% CI, 0.83–2.66, which was not statistically significant {140}. Neuro-imaging data from the Melbourne Women's Midlife Health Project of Australia show increased hippocampal activity in brains of young hormone users, compared with women of the same age and demographics who had never used hormone therapy {95}. The increased activity was associated with better memory. These scans suggest that if given early, estrogen has a beneficial effect on the hippocampus, an area that deteriorates in AD. Because of this misleading WHIMS report, women will stop their estrogen, and postmenopausal women will not start estrogen, therefore, missing the window of opportunity to have a significant impact on their lifetime risk of AD, which may be limited to the menopausal transition. This could result in millions more cases of this devastating disease.

HRT: Cardiovascular Results:

- Coronary Heart Disease (CHD)   HR = 1.29; 95% CI, 1.02–1.63
- Stroke   HR = 1.41; 95% CI 1.07–1.85
- Pulmonary Embolism   HR = 2.13; 95% CI, 1.39–3.25
- Total Deaths   HR = 0.98; 95% CI, 0.82–1.18

The second risk that triggered the stopping of the HRT arm of the WHI was coronary heart disease (CHD), with a 29 percent increase, or seven more events per 10,000 women per year. However, deaths from CVD were fewer in the *Prem-*

Pro users than the controls. When starting the study, these women were many years postmenopausal (average age 63), and had never used estrogen, so many already had cardiovascular risk factors.

Older women without menopausal symptoms were chosen for the WHI so that the placebo users would not develop hot flashes and drop out of the study. This data was not new because the HERS study, a secondary prevention tiral, had already shown an increased risk of heart disease in *PremPro* users {77}. The HERS study was stopped early, after four years, because there were more cardiovascular events in the hormone users than the controls. Nearly all of these events occurred in the first year of the HERS study RR = 1.52; 95% CI, 1.01–2.29. In the fourth and last year of the HERS study, the RR had dropped to 0.60, 95% CI, 0.36–0.98.

The Nurses Health Study, a very large study of over 100,000 nurses followed by questionnaire for over 20 years, in their mortality report of mostly *Premarin only* users, observed decreased death from heart disease and even cancer (see Table 6.1) {60}. In a retrospective secondary prevention trial of CVD mortality, Sullivan observed almost 100 percent survival for ten years in the *Premarin* users, compared to 60 percent in the non-users, (see Figure 8.5) {156}.

Osteoporosis

One of the positive findings in the WHI was that not only did hormone replacement decrease vertebral fractures, it also significantly reduces hip fracture.

FRACTURES:

- Hip   HR = 0.66; 95% CI, 0.45–0.98
- Vertebral   HR = 0.66; 95% CI, 0.44–0.99
- Other Fractures   HR = 0.77; 95% CI, 0.69–0.88
- Total Fractures   HR = 0.76; 95% CI, 0.69–0.85

SUMMARY OF RESULTS AT 5.2 YEARS

29%— ↑ in CVD (7 more events per 10,000 women per year)

26%— ↑ in Breast Cancer (8 more cancers per 10,000 women per year)

37%— ↓ in Colorectal Cancer (6 fewer cancers per 10,000 women per year)

34%— ↓ in Hip Fractures (6 fewer fractures per 10,000 women per year)

Dr. Leon Speroff has written that a theme has emereged from the epidemiologic confusion of the last few years {145}. It takes healthy tissue to allow an effective response to estrogen and maintenance of health. Experimental evidence indicates that as cells become involved with atheroscrlerosis and neurons become affected with the progression of Alzheimer's disease, beneficial response to estrogens decrease. Maximal benefit may require early onset of treatment, near the time of menopause.

Quality of Life

One area of little controversy is that hormone therapy has a beneficial impact on postmenopausal quality of life. Yet the WHI reported little benefit of HRT on quality of life. Why? WHI results do not apply to the majority of women prescribed hormone replacement therapy because in the WHI, the women selected were:

- Average age of 63 years
- 18 years distant from their menopause
- Had no significant symptoms (to avoid high dropout rate)

The WHI was a study of older women who were a relatively homogenous group with a good quality of life upon entry. It is very appropriate to question WHI conclusions with the usual HRT started at menopausal transition in women with postmenopausal symptoms. Women with significant menopausal symptoms were excluded from the WHI. Older women were chosen (mean age 63) who had never used estrogen, nor had hot flashes, so that the placebo users would not drop out of the WHI and "mess up their statistics". These older women who had never used estrogens already had increased risk for heart disease with some even having prior angioplasty or coronary by-pass surgery.

BENEFITS OF HRT IN 2004

- Relief of vasomotor symptoms
- Prevention of urogenital atrophy
- Alleviation of psychogenic manifestations
- Improved quality of life
- Prevention of osteoporosis
- Prevention of cardiovascular disease (CVD)
- Prevention of Alzheimer's Disease (AD)
- Reduction in macular degeneration of the retina
- Reduction in cataracts

Postmenopausal women need to continue estrogen therapy in adequate dosages for many years to achieve the maximum benefits. The lowest effective dosage for the shortest period of time is invalid since the benefits far exceed the risks; the WHI notwithstanding.

Summary of Conclusions

1. There is no new data in the Women's Health Initiative:
   a. The Collaborative Study on hormone factors in breast cancer showed a minimal increased risk after 5 years, RR = 1.115; 95% CI, 1.011–1.180
   b. The HERS study showed a ↑ RR of CVD of 1.29; 95% CI, 1.02–1.63
   c. The Cache County study shows that estrogen therapy initiated after age 60 increased AD, RR = 2.12, but decreased it by 83 percent when initiated at menopause transition.
2. The daily progestogen in the *PremPro* users decreased the estrogen receptors in coronary arteries and minimized the beneficial effect of estrogen.

3. The WHI was contrary to previous studies of estrogen therapy:
   a. Women with specific menopausal symptoms were excluded
   b. Older women were chosen (mean age 63) who had never used estrogen so that the placebo users would not drop out of the WHI
   c. These older women already had increased risk for heart disease and Alzheimer's Disease
   d. These older women were a homogenous group with a good quality of life upon entry—18 years distant from menopause
   e. It takes healthy tissue to allow an effective response to estrogen and maintenance of health
   f. As cells become involved with atherosclerosis and neurons become affected with AD, the beneficial response to estrogen decreases
   g. Maximal benefit of ERT may require early onset of treatment near the time of menopause
4. It is never too late to arrest the progression of osteoporosis and decrease the risk of fracture.

FIGURE 8.1—Cumulative Number Of Breast Cancers Diagnosed in 1000 Women {25}

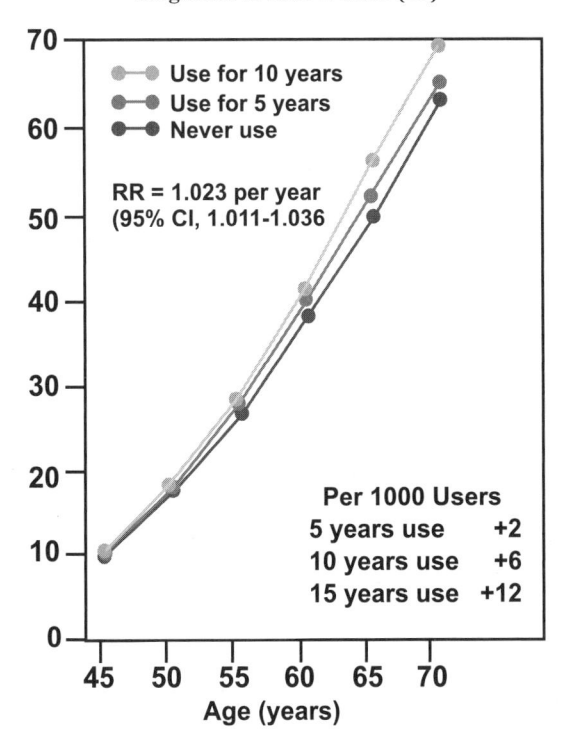

- Use for 10 years
- Use for 5 years
- Never use

RR = 1.023 per year
(95% CI, 1.011-1.036)

Per 1000 Users
5 years use   +2
10 years use +6
15 years use +12

Age (years)

FIGURE 8.2—Risk Estimates—Mortality / Survival—Estrogen Plus Progestogen

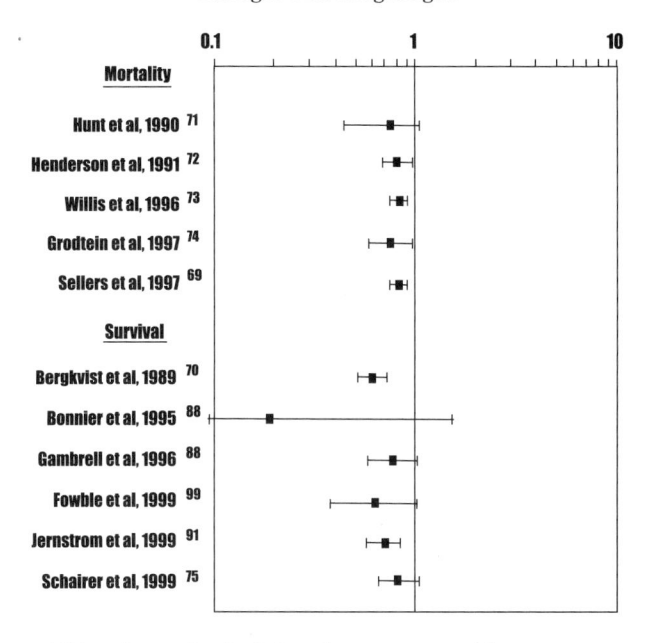

Mortality
- Hunt et al, 1990 [71]
- Henderson et al, 1991 [72]
- Willis et al, 1996 [73]
- Grodtein et al, 1997 [74]
- Sellers et al, 1997 [69]

Survival
- Bergkvist et al, 1989 [70]
- Bonnier et al, 1995 [88]
- Gambrell et al, 1996 [88]
- Fowble et al, 1999 [99]
- Jernstrom et al, 1999 [91]
- Schairer et al, 1999 [75]

Risk estimates for death from breast cancer and breast cancer survival: ever-users compared with never-users of hormone replacement therapy (estrogen plus progestogen). {12}

FIGURE 8.3—Risk Estimates For Incident Breast Cancer—Unopposed Estrogens

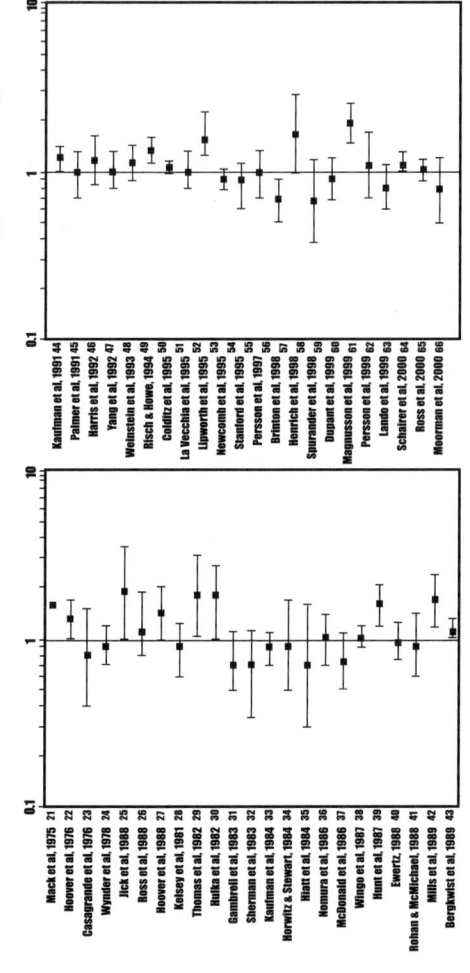

Risk estimates for incident breast cancer: ever-users compared with never-users of hormone replacement therapy—unopposed estrogens. {12}

FIGURE 8.4—Risk Estimates For Incident Breast Cancer—Estrogen Plus Progestogen

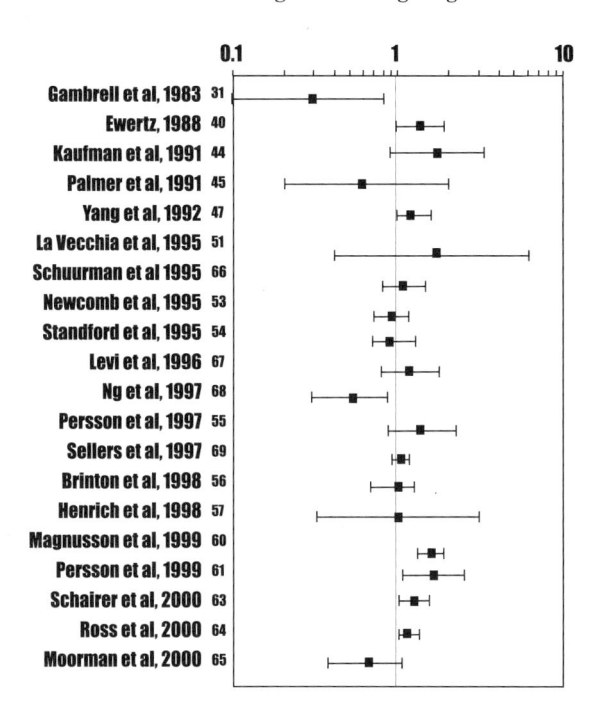

Gambrell et al, 1983	[31]
Ewertz, 1988	[40]
Kaufman et al, 1991	[44]
Palmer et al, 1991	[45]
Yang et al, 1992	[47]
La Vecchia et al, 1995	[51]
Schuurman et al 1995	[66]
Newcomb et al, 1995	[53]
Standford et al, 1995	[54]
Levi et al, 1996	[67]
Ng et al, 1997	[68]
Persson et al, 1997	[55]
Sellers et al, 1997	[69]
Brinton et al, 1998	[56]
Henrich et al, 1998	[57]
Magnusson et al, 1999	[60]
Persson et al, 1999	[61]
Schairer et al, 2000	[63]
Ross et al, 2000	[64]
Moorman et al, 2000	[65]

Risk estimates for incident breast cancer: ever-users compared with never-users of hormone replacement therapy (estrogen plus progestogen). {12}

FIGURE 8.5—Secondary Prevention Of CVD Mortality With Estrogen Therapy {156}

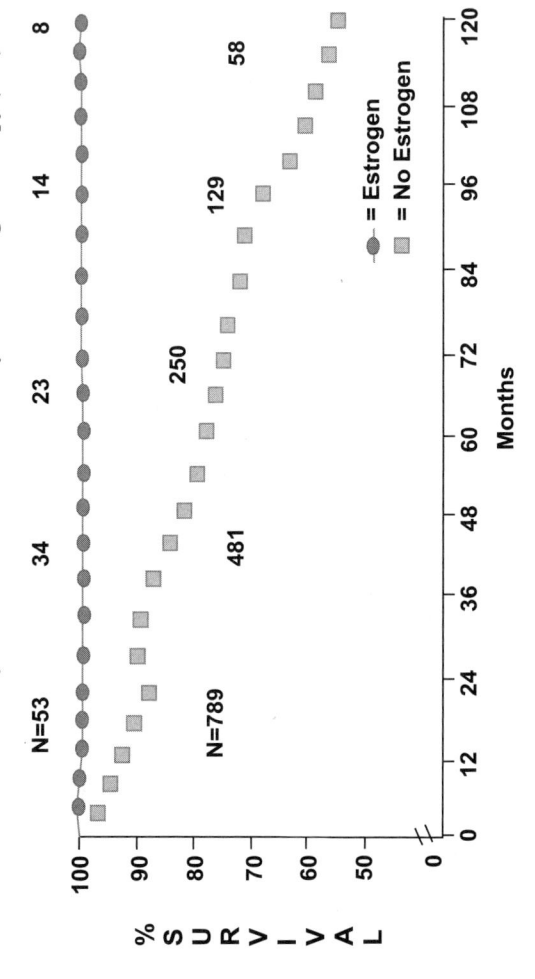

NOTES

SECTION 9: VAGINAL HORMONAL CYTOLOGY

Clinical Information

A patient's complaints of menopausal symptoms may be sufficient reason to begin estrogen replacement therapy (see Section 1). However, the vaginal smear is a good reflection of endogenous estrogen production.

With normal endogenous estrogen, there should be a high percentage, i.e. 15 to 30 percent, of superficial cells, which are cells with small pyknotic nuclei and a large amount of cytoplasm and the remaining cells should be of the intermediate types, larger nuclei with the nucleolus visible but still mostly cytoplasm. When parabasal cells (with a nucleus-to-cytoplasmic ratio of 50:50 or greater) are present on the vaginal smear, the patient usually has decreased estrogen production. If the vaginal smear is comprised of more than 50 percent parabasal cells, the patient is in a very hypoestrogenic state.

The physician can prepare the smear and read the vaginal hormonal cytology personally in order to provide instant information or send the vaginal smear to a cytology or pathology lab for a report of the maturation index (the percentage of superficial, intermediate, and parabasal cells). Most Pap smear reports now list an estrogen index.

Cytology Procedure

The smear is best taken from the lateral vaginal wall because it is usually more free of mucus and debris. A good instant stain for vaginal hormonal cytology is one percent pinacyanol. The pinacyanol chloride powder dye is obtained from the EastmanKodak Company, and the solution is made with one gram of dye in 100 cc of 90- to 95-percent alcohol (either ethanol or methanol).

After smearing the vaginal mucosa cells on a glass slide, a few drops of pinacyanol are applied and allowed to dry for one minute, then rinsed with ordinary tap water.

Slides are long-lasting, and the purple color can be freshened with drops of water or oil.

Fern Pattern Procedure

Another simple test used for estimation of estrogen production is the fern pattern of cervical mucus, although this can only be used with patients who have not had hysterectomies.

Mucus from the cervix is smeared onto a glass slide and allowed to dry for five minutes. If the fern pattern appears under the microscope, normal estrogen production is indicated, since the salts only crystallize with estrogen unopposed by progesterone.

During the normal ovulatory cycle, the fern pattern of cervical mucus increases from menses until ovulation and then rapidly disappears after ovulation due to progesterone. The fern pattern is also absent during pregnancy even though estrogen levels are high, because the high progesterone levels keep the cervical mucus from ferning.

Summary

Vaginal hormonal cytology and cervical mucus fern pattern cannot be used to diagnose menopause or to follow the effects of estrogen therapy, but these are adjunctive simple methods useful in evaluating patients with menopausal symptoms.

Estrogen replacement therapy should not be denied to severely symptomatic women on the basis of what appears to be a normal estrogen smear. Consideration should also be given to initiating hormone replacement in asymptomatic postmenopausal women with very hypoestrogenic vaginal smears. The latter group would possibly benefit from additional testing for osteoporosis risk by dual x-ray absorptiometry (DEXA).

Most symptomatic postmenopausal women need no additional testing other than the simple measures outlined above and the basic routine tests (see Section 13).

SECTION 10: PROGESTOGEN CHALLENGE TEST

Clinical Information

The progestogen challenge test should be administered to all postmenopausal women with intact uteri at annual evaluation. Included in this group are:

- Symptomatic women being evaluated for estrogen replacement therapy
- Estrogen-treated patients not already on progestogen therapy
- Asymptomatic postmenopausal women

The progesterone challenge test is the most reliable test for assessing potential estrogenic stimulation of the endometrium.

Not all postmenopausal women need estrogen replacement therapy, since many produce sufficient endogenous estrogens to remain asymptomatic and prevent the metabolic changes of estrogen deficiency in later life, such as:

- Atrophic vaginitis
- Osteoporosis
- Atherosclerosis
- Alzheimer's Disease

However, within this group may be those in greatest need of cyclic progestogen therapy to prevent endometrial hyperplasia, which may lead to adenocarcinoma.

Research

The progestogen challenge test was a concept evolved at Wilford Hall USAF Medical Center when it was recognized that the second highest incidence of endometrial cancer was observed in untreated postmenopausal women {46, 49}.

Original work on the progestogen challenge test has been confirmed by a prospective study using 100 mg of progesterone in oil given intramuscularly {49}. In a study of 30 asymptomatic postmenopausal women, five had withdrawal bleeding to the progestogen challenge and three of these (60 percent) had either adenomatous or atypical adenomatous hyperplasia. In the 25 subjects with no withdrawal bleeding, the endometrial histology was normal, mostly atrophic or inactive endometrium. There were no adenocarcinomas in either group; and, although the number of subjects was small, the difference between the two groups was statistically significant ($P \leq 0.001$).

In the second phase of this study in which 10 patients with known adenomatous hyperplasia were tested, the progestogen challenge test resulted in withdrawal bleeding in nine (90 percent), confirming the effectiveness of this test in detecting abnormal endometrial pathology.

The conclusion was that the progestogen challenge test was a reliable screening test for detecting women at greater risk for developing endometrial hyperplasia or adenocarcinoma. Other studies have confirmed that the progestogen challenge test is a reliable test for identifying women at high risk for endometrial cancer.

In a study in which the progestogen challenge test was given to 292 elderly women (mean age = 71.2 years), 14 (4.8 percent) had either spotting or bleeding {119}. Endometrial biopsies revealed significant pathology in three of these women: one endometrial cancer, one hyperplasia, and one chronic endometritis. Atrophic endometrium was found in eight, a proliferative endometrium in one, and an insufficient sample in two.

Procedure

The progestogen challenge test is performed by administering a 13-day course of progestogen (either medroxyprogesterone acetate 10 mg or norethindrone acetate 5 mg) to postmenopausal women with intact uteri (see Section #17). If a positive response occurs, as manifested by withdrawal bleeding, progestogens should be continued for 13 days each month for as long as withdrawal bleeding follows. If there is a negative response, it is recommended that the progestogen challenge be repeated each year in asymptomatic postmenopausal women not taking hormones.

Annual endometrial biopsies are not necessary in estrogen-progestogen users (see Section 11). Because of the benefits of added progestogen on the bones and the breast (see Sections 5 and 23}, this hormone should be continued in estrogen users, regardless of withdrawal bleeding.

NOTES

SECTION 11: ENDOMETRIAL BIOPSY

Clinical Information

Women receiving unopposed estrogen therapy should have annual endometrial biopsies. Post-menopausal women with any abnormal bleeding or responding by bleeding to the progestogen challenge test should have one of the following:
- An extensive endometrial biopsy
- Ultrasound
- Formal diagnostic dilatation and curettage (D&C)
- Hysteroscopy

Perimenopausal women who have irregular menses should have each of the following:
- Extensive endometrial sampling
- Pap smear
- Cervical biopsy, after Schiller's stain or colposcopically-directed if smear is abnormal
- Endocervical curettage
- Bimanual examination

An exception to these in estrogen-progestogen users is in situations in which bleeding occurs on or after day 11 of progestogen therapy. In these cases, no evaluation is necessary since the histology has been shown to be predominantly secretory {112}. Because of the recent appearance of several cases of endometrial cancer after years of amenorrhea in patients using continuous combined estrogen-progestogen therapy, any spotting or breakthrough bleeding after the first year of therapy should be promptly investigated (see Section 22).

Endometrial Evaluation Methods

The traditional method for evaluating the endometrium has been diagnostic D&C. However, hospitalization for a D&C, even on an outpatient basis, has disadvantages including:
- Increased anesthetic risk
- Additional expense
- Delay in diagnosis

These problems can be avoided by a properly performed clinic or office curettage, using the Pipelle Endometrial Suction Curette. The endometrial cavity should be sampled twice if much tissue is extracted. Frequently, the endometrial Pipelle can be utilized without a tenaculum or without sounding the uterus. This process will yield as much information as a outpatient D&C.

Although there is patient discomfort with the office procedure, the discomfort may be minimized by gentleness and a careful explanation of each step. Discomfort can also be reduced by placing four-percent *Xylocaine Viscous* on a small cotton-tipped applicator in the endocervical canal for three to five minutes. Paracervical blocks can also be performed; however, these may be more painful than the procedure itself.

Other satisfactory endometrial evaluation methods include:
- Curity Isaacs Endometrial Cell Sampler
- The Vabra Aspirator
- The Milex Endometrial Cannula
- Randall or Novak Suction biopsy

Summary

Endometrial biopsies are desirable before beginning estrogen replacement therapy but may only be necessary for those who respond to the progestogen challenge test by bleeding (see Section 10).

Progestogen challenge tests were performed in the Wilford Hall USAF Medical Center studies {46}. Consequently, most of the endometrial cancers in estrogen-progestogen users were probably already present from the unopposed estrogens before the progestogen was added {49}. If the progestogen challenge test is utilized as directed, patients with a negative response to the test (no withdrawal bleeding) do not need an endometrial biopsy. The progestogen challenge test is just as reliable as endometric ultrasound {62}.

In addition, it is easier to perform the biopsy if the patient returns on the first or second day of withdrawal bleeding. In approximately 10 to 15 percent of postmenopausal women, the cervix is so stenotic that endometrial biopsies are difficult to perform in the office; and withdrawal bleeding dilates the cervix slightly, which facilitates sounding and performing the biopsy in the clinic.

NOTES

SECTION 12: OSTEOPOROSIS DETECTION METHODS

Types of Methods Available
There are at least four methods of screening women to determine bone loss. These include:
- Regular x-ray
- Single and dual x-ray absorptiometry
- Quantitative computed axial tomography (QCT) scan
- Dual energy x-ray absorptiometry (DXA)
- Ultrasound

Regular X-Ray
Regular x-ray of the bones can reveal osteoporosis. However, before osteoporosis can be detected on regular x-ray, a loss of 30 to 40 percent of total bone mass must have occurred. This is a fairly late stage of the disease.

Newer and better methods reveal lesser amounts of bone loss to allow earlier detection and prompt treatment of the condition.

Single and Dual X-Ray Absorptiometry
Photon absorptiometry was developed in the early 1960s while researchers were looking for a method to determine the effect of gravity on bones (particularly, the effect on astronauts). This technique detects small amounts of bone loss, allowing early diagnosis and treatment of osteoporosis. Another advantage is the method's very low radiation exposure, about 1/100 that of standard x-rays.

Single photon absorptiometry is used to measure bone mass in the radius using radioactive iodine (I-131). The amount of radiation that passes through the bone is measured by a detector positioned above the arm, thus determining the thickness of the bone.

Dual photon absorptiometry (DPA) uses radioactive gadolinium (Gd-153) as the radiation source. The DPA has been substituted by the DEXA that, instead of using a radioactive source of energy, uses an x-ray beam. It measures bone thickness in the vertebrae (AP or lateral), hip, or femur. Total body calcium can also be measured with this technique. The

latest improvement in this method is its detection of bone density of the total body or any part of it, such as:
- Cervical area
- Thoracic or lumbar spine
- Arms
- Legs
- Pelvis
- Ribs

Computers are used with these methods to aid in determining the percent of bone present compared to standards (young-normals) and bone densities found in patients matched for age, sex, and height. The results are plotted on a graph, with the patient's bone thickness or bone mineral density (BMD) on the Y axis and age on the X axis. Standard deviations (SD) are provided for an accurate mode of diagnosis and are represented as every line under the normal mean.

The results are given as a percentage of normal, young women and percentage of age-matched. The standards of bone mass that should be present were worked out at the Mayo Clinic and the University of Wisconsin.

The computer-generated and printed report provides the physician with information about bone mass, including:
- T-Score: bone density of the individual compared to young, normal controls
- Z-Score: bone density compared to age, weight, height, and race matched controls

Evaluating osteoporosis T-Score is important as it gives the true evaluation of the bone loss in that individual, compared to a young individual. Fracture rates increase by two for each drop of T-Score of one deviation. Up to two standard deviation is called osteopenia. More than two standard deviations diagnoses osteoporosis.

The report also indicates on a graph whether the degree of the patient's risk for fracture is:
- Normal
- Mild
- Moderate
- Severe

Quantitative Computed Axial Tomography (QCT)

A QCT scan was the most accurate measurement of bone until x-ray densitometry was developed. The QCT scan is more expensive; and since it uses x-rays as the radiation source, the amount of radiation exposure is considerably higher than that of dual radiation absorptiometry, 13 to 20 times higher.

In young women whose ovaries have been removed, a QCT scan can detect bone loss in the spine very early, as soon as two to four months after surgery. The method is, therefore, very useful in research on osteoporosis, but it is not necessary in evaluating patients for estrogen therapy.

Need for Bone Measurements

Most women do not need any of these osteoporosis screening methods. But for medical researchers, these tests are essential to determine:
- Dosages of estrogen
- The need for supplemental calcium
- Additions of other therapies, e.g.,:
  - Vitamin D
  - Progestogens
  - Bisphosphonates

These tests may also be useful in following patients who already have osteoporosis to ensure that its progression has been stopped with the present therapy.

If patients will seek medical evaluation for estrogen deficiency and physicians will treat patients for estrogen deficiency, osteoporosis can be prevented.

It is known that oral therapy with 0.625 mg of conjugated estrogens will prevent osteoporosis in more than 90 percent of postmenopausal women. Active clinical research is being conducted on other types of estrogens to determine the dosages necessary to prevent osteoporosis. Now that 0.5 mg of micronized estradiol is available and 0.625 mg of estropipate is being promoted by different pharmaceutical companies, concern must be expressed that these lower dosages of estrogen are not preventive for the majority of postmenopausal women over the long term (see Section 5).

Biochemical Bone Markers

The urinary biochemical bone markers, pyridinium crosslinks and telopeptides, may be helpful in monitoring bone loss in estrogen users. Bone markers are not predictive of bone loss in untreated postmenopausal women, nor can they be used to diagnose osteoporosis {39}. Up to 10 percent of postmenopausal estrogen users may be losing bone in spite of adequate estrogen replacement. Where urinary bone markers may be useful is in monitoring estrogen users to be sure their bone mineral density is being maintained. When these bone markers are elevated, which may indicate higher bone loss than replacement, bone density studies should be done to assess the bone adequately.

Other agents, such as SERMS, calcitonin and parathormone are used to treat osteoporosis since estrogens are approved only for prevention of osteoporosis. The bisphosphonates, and perhaps the other approved agents, can be added to estrogen to prevent further bone loss.

Currently bone markers are used primarily in research since DXA scans are more accurate in predicting osteoporosis.

Osteoporosis Screening Clinics

Using urinary markers and bone densities estrogen users can be screened to see if they need other modalities of therapy such as bisphophonates or parathormone.

A number of osteoporosis screening clinics are springing up across the U.S. These are beneficial because they are increasing public awareness of osteoporosis.

BMD may be lost due to causes other than estrogen deficiency (e.g., thyroid or parathyroid abnormalities), long-term prednisone therapy, or endocrinopathies in which cortisol is increased. Patients who have undergone gastrointestinal surgeries, i.e., ileostomies, which remove the area where calcium absorption takes place, or who have kidney function impairment (which nullifies vitamin D_3 activity, 1.25 DHC) are subject to bone loss also.

Most women do not need to be screened for osteoporosis and only need to be treated with estrogens if they are estrogen-deficient. However, more than just screening techniques (x-ray densitometry) should be used to follow hormonal response in patients with bone loss.

Although screening is not seen as cost-effective initially, it is in the long-term because osteoporosis is a major public health problem affecting more than 10 million Americans {Ref 115} at an annual cost of $10 to 12 billion. For this reason, prevention is the best way to avoid osteoporosis. It is far better to prevent bone loss than it is to treat osteoporosis.

Who Should Be Screened?

There are certain known factors that increase the risk for osteoporosis {115,125}. It is not unreasonable to screen women who have multiple risk factors, including:

- White or Asian heritage
- A positive family history of osteoporosis
- Low calcium intake (lifelong)
- Early menopause
- Ovaries removed at a young age
- Sedentary lifestyle
- Alcohol abuse
- High salt intake
- Cigarette smoking
- High caffeine intake
- High protein intake
- High phosphate intake
- Diseases such as hyperthyroidism
- Certain drugs, e.g., such as steroids

NOTES

SECTION 13: LABORATORY AND TESTS FOR EARLY CANCER DETECTION

Basic Tests

There are a number of basic tests that should be performed when evaluating patients for estrogen replacement therapy. These include:
- Blood pressure
- Electrolytes
- Liver function
- Renal function
- Enzymes
- Complete blood count (CBC)
- Blood indices
- Platelet count
- Thyroxine
- Urinalysis

Add as needed:
- FSH
- Estradiol
- Testosterone
- Free Testosterone

Additional tests should be obtained if indicated from the history. For example, with a history of non-traumatic thromboembolic disease, the following should be added to the platelet count:
- Prothrombin time
- Partial thromboplastin time
- Antithrombin III

Consideration should be given to fractionalization of cholesterol into HDL and LDL, since LDL cholesterol may be increased after menopause. However, if total cholesterol is below 200 mg/dL and triglycerides are below 150 mg/dL, it is not necessary to fractionate cholesterol levels into HDL and LDL.

These routine tests should be repeated after six months of estrogen therapy and repeated approximately every one to two years thereafter during estrogen therapy.

Follow-up Tests

Annual tests that should be performed include:
- Pap smear in patients with uteri
- Bimanual examination
- Rectal examination

Semiannual tests that should be performed include:
- Blood pressure
- Hemoglobin
- Breast examination

Mammography

Any abnormality of the breasts requires prompt evaluation by mammography and/or direct biopsy. Likewise, any changes in mammary tissue require immediate evaluation. Breast self-examination should be taught to patients and recommended monthly. Semiannual breast exams should be done by the physician, more often if palpable abnormalities are present.

The American Cancer Society's guidelines on mammography should be followed. For the normally palpable breast, mammograms should be performed as follows:
- A baseline mammogram should be obtained at age 40
- Mammogram should be obtained annually after age 40

A controversy has arisen over the cost-effectiveness of mammography screening in women ages 40 to 50 at the U.S. Department of Health and Human Services {50}. However, the American Cancer Society, the American College of Radiology, and ACOG still recommend it; and it has been invaluable in the author's practice.

Estrogen therapy does not increase the risk for breast cancer (see Section 23), but postmenopausal women are reaching the age at which the incidence of breast cancer continuously increases.

Tests for Colon and Rectal Cancer

Colon and rectal cancers are the second most frequent cancers in women, i.e.,11 percent of all female cancers, and the third leading killer from cancer in women (10 percent of all female cancer deaths). The American Cancer Society estimated that there would be 73,470 new cases of colon and rectal cancers in females in the U.S. during 2005, resulting in the death of 25,750 women from these malignancies {79}

The American Cancer Society recommendations for early detection of colon and rectal cancers include:
- Digital rectal examination annually at age 40
- Stool guaiac slide test annually at age 50
- Sigmoidoscopy or colonoscopy every three to five years at age 50

Reduction in Colon Cancer

The most recent benefit shown for hormone replacement therapy is the 30- to 40-percent reduction in colon cancer. Sex steroid hormones modify hepatic cholesterol production and alter bile acid concentration. Increased concentrations of bile acids have long been thought to be important in human colon cancer carcinogenesis. In animal studies, bile acids promote tumors. It has been suggested that exogenous estrogens and progestogen may reduce the secretion of bile acids {101}.

Studies are now confirming that hormone replacement therapy, either estrogens alone or in combination with progestogen, significantly reduce the risk of colon cancer RR = 0.54; 95% CI, 0.36 to 0.81 {109}. Overall, postmenopausal hormone use was associated with a 30 percent reduction in colon cancer for ever-use, and a 46 percent reduction for recent use.

In a study of 422,373 postmenopausal women, the risk of colon cancer in estrogen users was reduced to RR = 0.71 95% CI, 0.61 to 0.83 {172}. With 11 or more years of estrogen use, the reduction was RR = 0.54; 95% CI, 0.39 to 0.76. Similar results have been seen in the WHI study—RR = 0.63; 95% CI, 0.45–0.95 {131}.

Diagnosis

The diagnosis of menopause can usually be made by history and physical examination, including vaginal hormonal cytology and the progestogen challenge test. If still uncertain, the best single laboratory test is serum FSH.

Postmenopausally, serum FSH and LH values are markedly elevated, with FSH in the range of 75 to 200 mIU/mL and LH in the range of 60 to 90 mIU/mL. Within a year after menses ceases, serum FSH may increase as much as 13-fold, while LH rises approximately threefold. After a further rise in both FSH and LH during early postmenopausal years, there is a gradual decline with age.

Thirty years after menopausal onset, serum gonadotropin levels are only 40 to 50 percent of the maximum reached. However, these levels are still much higher than those found during reproductive years. Serum FSH is more reliable for diagnosis of menopause, since it usually rises more quickly and to higher levels than LH. Also, the midcycle LH surge in ovulating women could be mistaken for a postmenopausal level. If the serum FSH is above 30 mIU/mL, that patient is estrogen-deficient and should be started on replacement therapy.

Serum estrogen levels are unreliable for diagnosis of menopause, since the range of normal is so wide. Serum estradiol varies from five to 25 pg/mL after menopause and from 25 to 75 pg/mL in the follicular phase in women of reproductive age. Even total urinary estrogens cannot be used, since postmenopausal values are five to 15 micrograms per 24 hours compared to 10 to 25 micrograms per 24 hours during the follicular phase in ovulatory women. Estrogen levels in peri-menopausal women should not be used for diagnosis. Peaks and valleys occur in estrogen levels as ovarian function decreases. FSH levels can be used since high levels of FSH indicate ovarian failure. Testosterone and free testosterone levels can be performed especially if a patient has symptoms of fatigue, depression and/or loss of libido.

SECTION 14: ORAL ESTROGENS

Clinical Information

When the uterus is present, the patient with menopausal symptoms should be prescribed estrogens and progestogens after proper evaluation (see Section 13) and in the absence of contraindications (see Section 30).

Dosages

Cyclic therapy is usually recommended in order to minimize side effects. However, continuous estrogen therapy is just as safe as long as the estrogen is opposed by a progestogen. Conjugated estrogens at 0.625 mg or equivalent dosages of other natural estrogens (see Table 14.1) can be given according to the calendar from the first through the 25th of the month. The progestogen should be added during the last 13 days of estrogen therapy, from the 13th through the 25th (see Table 17.1). If symptoms recur on the days off estrogens, continuous therapy can be used as long as the estrogen is opposed by a progestogen.

Although lower dosages are available, 0.625 mg of conjugated estrogens is the dosage that has been shown to prevent osteoporosis in more than 90 percent of postmenopausal women. Since prevention of osteoporosis is the major goal of estrogen replacement therapy, this is the lowest dosage that should be used.

If symptoms such as hot flushes persist after two to three months of estrogen therapy, the estrogen dosage can be increased from 0.625 to 0.9 or 1.25 mg of conjugated estrogens. Doses above 1.25 mg are rarely necessary to relieve menopausal symptoms. It is more advisable to add an androgen (see Section 16) than continually increase the estrogen dose.

Exceptions

There are two exceptions to the normal 0.625 mg estrogen dosage. These are for women who:

- Have had surgical menopause during their reproductive years
- Have osteoporosis

Women with surgical menopause whose ovaries are removed during reproductive years usually require higher dosages of conjugated estrogens (e.g., 1.25 mg) to relieve menopausal symptoms. However, after one to two years, this dose can usually be reduced to 0.625 mg.

Women with osteoporosis also need a higher dosage; 1.25 mg of conjugated estrogen is recommended to reduce fracture rates.

Summary

It is sometimes more difficult to evaluate patients who have had hysterectomies and to initiate proper estrogen therapies for them. If bilateral oophorectomies are also performed during reproductive years, estrogen therapy should be initiated soon afterwards. Dosages of 1.25 mg conjugated estrogens are often required for prevention of symptoms.

When ovaries are preserved, menopausal symptoms are commonly delayed until the time of natural menopause. However, after a hysterectomy, the ovaries may not continue to function fully until the expected age of natural menopause. Patients presenting with obvious vasomotor symptoms and/or atrophic vaginitis should be started on cyclic estrogen therapy with 0.625 mg of conjugated estrogens from the first through the 25th of each month.

For women who have had hysterectomies with conservation of ovaries, and who have minimal symptoms, vaginal hormonal cytology and serum FSH may aid diagnosis. To prevent osteoporosis, estrogen therapy can be instituted when hormonal evidence of menopause exists. In addition, from the 13th through the 25th of each month, cyclic progestogens should be added to the hormone therapy for additional protection of the bones (see Section 5) and the breasts (see Section 23).

TABLE 14.1: ORAL ESTROGENS

Name	Brand Name	Manufacturer	Available Dosage Forms	Usual Maintenance Dose
Conjugated Estrogens	Cenestin	Duramed	0.3,0.625,0.9,1.25mg tablet	0.625 mg PO qd
Conjugated Estrogens	Premarin	Wyeth	0.3,0.625,0.9,1.25,2.5mg tablet	0.625 mg PO qd
Esterified Estrogens	Menest	Monarch	0.3,0.625,1.25,2.5mg tablet	0.625 mg PO qd
Esterified Estrogens	Estratab	Solvay	0.625,1.25mg	0.625 mg
Estradiol	Estrace	Warner-Chilcott	0.5,1,2-mg tablet	1–2 mg PO qd
Estradiol	Gynodiol	Novavax	0.5,1.5, 2-mg tablet	1.5 mg PO qd
Estropipate	Ogen	Watson	0.75,1.5,3.0 tablet	1.5 mg PO qd

TABLE 14.2: ESTROGEN–PROGESTOGEN

Name	Brand Name	Manufacturer	Available Dosage Forms	Usual Maintenance Dose
Conjugated estrogens/ Medroxy-progesterone acetate	Premphase	Wyeth	0.625mg tablet (14 tabs) 0.625mg/5mg tablet (14 tabs)	0.625 1–14; 15–28 0.625mg/5mg PO qd
Conjugated estrogens/ Medroxy-progesterone acetate	Prempro	Wyeth	0.625mg/5mg tablet 0.625mg/2.5mg tablet 0.45mg/1.5mg tablet 0.3mg/1.5mg tablet	0.625mg/5mg
Estradiol/norethindrone acetate	Activella	Pharmacia	1mg/0.5mg tablet	1mg/0.5mg PO qd
Estradiol/norgestimate	Prefest	Duramed	1mg/0.09mg tablet	1mg/0.09mg PO qd
Ethinyl estradiol/norethindrone acetate	FemHRT 1/5 FemHRT 0.5/2.5	Warner Chilcott	5-mg/1-mg tablet 2.5-mg/0.5-mg tablet	5 mg/1 mg PO qd

SECTION 15: NON-ORAL ESTROGENS

Estrogen Vaginal Cream

Estrogen vaginal cream is the longest available and probably the most useful of the non-oral estrogens. In creams, estrogens are well-absorbed through the vaginal mucosa so that good systemic levels are obtained as well as the local beneficial effects. Vaginal creams probably provide the quickest response and subsequent relief of symptoms of atrophic vaginitis, such as:

- Vaginal irritation
- Pruritus
- Vaginal dryness
- Dyspareunia

One common course of treatment is to apply *Premarin* vaginal cream, 1g daily (see Table 15.1) or *Estrace Vaginal Cream*. Usually, oral estrogens are started simultaneously. After two weeks of double therapy, the maintenance dosage of the vaginal cream can often be reduced to three times weekly or can be entirely eliminated.

However, some patients on oral estrogens may continue to require estrogen vaginal cream for maintenance of the vaginal mucosa. Also, some women may not respond adequately to oral estrogens alone, developing dryness or pruritus of the vagina while on therapy. Instead of increasing the oral estrogen dosage, these women frequently benefit more from the addition of estrogen vaginal cream to the therapeutic routine.

Use of oral estrogens has been questioned because of portal absorption and liver metabolism as well as the risk of cholelithiasis. With the first liver-pass, hepatic enzymatic changes may be induced that alter various biochemical parameters. Oral therapy may result in estrogen being delivered directly into hepatic tissue via the portal circulation. This could possibly result in changes in the rates of synthesis of certain hepatically derived proteins and globulins, such as:

- Renin substrate
- Cortisol-binding globulin (CBG)
- Sex hormone-binding globulin (SHBG)
- Antithrombin III

Most of these changes are minor and may not be clinically significant.

Non-oral routes of administration deliver the estrogen directly into the systemic circulation and, thus, may cause less marked changes in hepatic biosynthesis because the portal system is by-passed. However, at least one of the benefits of oral therapy, the increase in HDL cholesterol, may be delayed by non-oral administration. Apparently, the first liver-pass induces this antiatherogenic lipoprotein more quickly.

Saturated Vaginal Rings

Silastic vaginal rings can be saturated with sex steroids, releasing fairly constant amounts of estrogen and/or progestogen into peripheral blood. Whether this method will be widely accepted by patients remains to be determined, but cyclic therapy with the natural steroids (estradiol and progesterone) can be provided through the vaginal mucosa.

An estradiol vaginal ring containing 2 mg of estradiol (*Estring*—Pharmacia) has been used for treatment of atrophic vaginitis. There is little to no systemic absorption, so it is intended for local use only. One ring will last for 90 days. There is improvement in vaginal mucosal epithelium after 12 weeks, and the vaginal pH is restored to normal.

Another vaginal ring (*Femring*—Warner Chilcott) is designed for systemic absorption (like the patches) to treat moderate to severe vasomotor symptoms of menopause, and vulvar to vaginal atrophy. It is available for systemic as well as local delivery of estradiol. The ring is inserted every three months and is available in two doses: Estradiol Acetate. 0.05 mg/day and 0.1 mg/day.

In contrast to oral micronized estradiol, vaginal estradiol:

- Provides a low estrone-to-estradiol ratio
- Does not induce a high postmedication estrogen peak

- Reaches the peripheral circulation without passing the enterohepatic circulation

Estradiol Subcutaneous Pellets

Subcutaneous implantation of 17β-estradiol pellets, the principal human estrogen, has been available for more than 65 years. It was, however, taken off the market by the FDA in 1980 for lack of efficacy and safety studies. Pellets are available under USP approval and can be obtained from the compounding pharmacies. (Table 15.2)

The main use of estradiol pellets has been by patients who could not use oral estrogens because of a lack of response, or because of side effects associated with oral estrogens. Estradiol pellets have been shown to be very effective in relieving menopausal symptoms, including:
- Hot flushes (or flashes)
- Insomnia
- Dyspareunia

Side effects, which occur in five to eight percent of oral estrogen users, are diminished in those who use pellets because of the use of the major ovarian estrogen.

When combined with subcutaneous testosterone pellets, estradiol implants are particularly effective in treating psychosexual problems such as loss of libido and anorgasmia, which may not respond to estrogen alone (58, 154). Estradiol pellets provide more normal estrone-to-estradiol ratios than oral estrogens and also provide more constant estrogen levels than any parenteral form of estrogen administration.

Transdermal Estradiol

The transdermal system of estrogen replacement therapy is another form of non-oral administration. This system has been shown to be clinically effective in relieving menopausal symptoms. Comparative studies indicate that the transdermal system provides more normal estrone-to-estradiol ratios than oral estrogens.

Transdermal estradiol elicited many of the desirable actions of estrogen while avoiding the pharmacologic effects of oral estrogens on hepatic proteins (19). The patches are placed on the skin at 8:00 a.m. Monday and 8:00 p.m. Thursday, since estradiol levels are effective for three and one-half days. (Table 15.3) Patches should be used continuously, since symptoms may return when patches are removed because of rapidly falling estradiol levels.

Other transdermal estrogens available in different doses 0.025, 0.05, 0.075 and 0.1 mg are once-a-week *Climara*, and twice-a-week *Vivelle* and *Alora*, which are smaller. Generic patches are also available. Skin irritation seems to be less, although the patch is left on the skin for a longer duration. These matrix patches have no alcohol (acid alcohol is a primary skin irritant).

Although there are few or no undesirable effects with transdermal systems, endometrial proliferation is normal and an oral progestogen must be given for 10 to 13 days. Transdermal estradiol takes longer to produce a rise in HDL cholesterol than do oral estrogens {148}. Over the long-term, patches should be just as protective from atherosclerotic heart disease, especially with the 0.1 mg estradiol dosage.

A combination estradiol/progestogen patch is available in two different dosages (Table 15.4). Both have the same dosage of estradiol, 0.05 mg, but different dosages of the progestogen, norethindrone acetate, either 0.14 mg or 0.25 mg. These different dosages have the advantage that if breakthrough bleeding should persist beyond 3 or 4 months on the lower dosage, it can be changed to Combipatch 50/250.

TABLE 15.1: ESTROGEN VAGINAL CREAMS AND RINGS

Generic Name	Brand Name	Manufacturer	Available Dosage Forms	Usual Maintenance Dose
Conjugated estrogens	Premarin	Wyeth	0.625mg per g vaginal cream	1g 1-3×/wk
Estradiol	Estring Vaginal Ring	Pharmacia	2-mg vaginal insert	Replace ring every 90 d
Estradiol	Vagifem	Pharmacia	25-mcg vaginal Tablet	1 tab 2×/wk
Estropipate	Ogen	Pharmacia	1.5-mg per g vaginal cream	2–4 g 1-3×/wk
Micronized estradiol	Estrace	Warner Chilcott	0.01% cream	1 g 1–3×/wk
Estradiol	Femring	Warner Chilcott	0.05mg, 0.1mg	every 90 days

TABLE 15.2: PARENTERAL INTRAMUSCULAR ESTROGENS

Generic Name	Brand Name	Manufacturer	Available Dosage Forms	Usual Maintenance Dose
Estradiol cypionate	Depo-Estradiol	Pharmacia	5mg/mL injection	1–5-mg IM q 3–4wk
Estradiol valerate	Delestrogen	Monarch	10mg/mL, 20mg/mL, 40mg/mL injection	10–20mg IM q 4wk
Estradiol Pellet	Estradiol Pellet	Various Pharmacies	25 mg	25–50 mg q 5–6 mos

TABLE 15.3: TRANSDERMAL ESTROGENS

Generic Name	Brand Name	Manufacturer	Available Dosage Forms	Usual Maintenance Dose	Comments
Estradiol	Alora	Watson	0.05, 0.075, 0.1mg per 24/h patch	0.05mg per 24/h patch	Twice a week
Estradiol	Climara	Berlex	0.025, 0.0375, 0.05, 0.06, 0.075, 0.1mg	0.05mg per 24/h patch	Once a week
Estradiol	Esclim	Women First	0.025, 0.0375, 0.05, 0.06, 0.075, 0.1mg per 24/h patch	0.05mg per 24/h patch	Twice a week
Estradiol	Estraderm	Novartis	0.05, 0.1mg per 24/h patch	0.05mg per 24/h patch	Twice a week
Estradiol	Vivelle	Novartis	0.025, 0.0375, 0.05, 0.075, 0.1mg per 24/h	0.05mg per 24/h patch	Twice a week
Estradiol	Vivelle dot	Novartis	0.025, 0.0375, 0.05, 0.075, 0.1mg per 24/h patch	0.05mg per 24/h patch	Twice a week

TABLE 15.4: TRANSDERMAL ESTROGEN-PROGESTOGEN

Generic Name	Brand Name	Manufacturer	Available Dosage Forms	Comment
Estradiol/Norethindrone Acetate	Combipatch 50/140	Novartis	0.05/0.140 mg per 24/h patch	Twice a week
	Combipatch 50/250	Novartis	0.05/0.250 mg per 24/h patch	Twice a week

SECTION 16: ANDROGENS

Clinical Information

Estrogens relieve most of the menopausal symptoms. However, it sometimes becomes necessary to add androgens to hormone replacement therapy. Up to 75 percent of estrogen production is lost after menopause, but up to 50 percent of androgen production can also be lost when ovaries cease to function or are surgically removed. If symptoms persist, it is best to add a low dose of androgen to the estrogen replacement regimen than to continue increasing the estrogen dosage beyond 1.25 mg of conjugated estrogens (see Table 16.1).

Potential benefits of androgens include alleviation of:
- Hot flushes (or flashes)
- Lethargy
- Endogenous depression
- Kraurosis vulvae (with use of one- to two- percent testosterone cream)
- Nocturia and incontinence
- Fibrocystic disease of the breast
- Headaches (migrainoid)
- Fatigue

Although estrogens will alleviate both hot flushes and genital atrophy, the addition of an androgen will help overcome fatigue. In patients with breast cancer who are usually denied the use of estrogens, androgens may be used. Androgens alone may be helpful to relieve vasomotor symptoms and improve the psyche. However, they are of little value in treatment of genital atrophy and probably do not prevent osteoporosis in the dosages that can be used.

Some postmenopausal women complain of hirsutism before any hormone replacement. This is probably due to a relative imbalance of endogenous estrogens and androgens where estrogen levels decrease more than testosterone levels. Typically manifested by an increase in upper lip hair or small moustache, this usually lessens after estrogen replacement.

Androgen therapy can aggravate:
- Pre-existing hirsutism
- Acne
- Skin oiliness

If there are good results from the androgen, but aggravation of hirsutism or acne, reducing the androgen dosage and/or increasing the estrogen dosage may help. Spironolactone at 25 mg four times daily may also be added to the estrogen-androgen combination so that the benefits of the androgen can be continued.

Research

In one study, patients experienced relief of hot flushes with non-oral therapies {58} as follows:
- Ninety-six percent with estradiol pellets
- Eighty-nine percent with estradiol pellets plus testosterone
- Fifty-five percent with testosterone alone
- Sixteen percent with placebo

Estrogen alone gave less benefit than estrogen-androgen pellets, when used for:
- Increasing feelings of well-being
- Improving libido
- Relieving endogenous depression
- Lessening migrainoid headaches

In postmenopausal women, androgens added to estrogen replacement commonly improved problems with:
- Libido
- Sexual response
- Anorgasmia

An increase in libido occurred {58} in:
- More than 65 percent of those treated with androgens
- 12.3 percent of those receiving estrogens
- Only 1.8 percent of those taking the placebo

In a study in which 76 women received pellet implants of 50 mg estradiol, a combination of 50 mg estradiol and 100 mg testosterone, or placebo every six months, only those on the combination estrogen-androgen experienced a decided increase in sexual response and frequency of coitus {153, 154}. The addition of testosterone implants also increased the frequency and intensity of orgasmic responses.

Recommendations

Available forms of androgen and estrogen-androgen combinations are found in Table 16.1.

ORAL THERAPY

Estratest or *Estratest H.S.* is well tolerated. Therapy should be cyclic from the first through the 25th of the month to minimize side effects, and a progestogen should be added from the 13th through the 25th of the month. Although androgens may suppress the endometrium slightly, most patients on estrogen-androgen combinations will have withdrawal menses from the progestogen challenge test.

INJECTABLES

Depo-Testadiol 1 cc IM will usually relieve symptoms for four weeks.

SUBCUTANEOUS PELLETS

Estradiol pellets are available in the U.S. from certain pharmacies. Testosterone pellets are the only available form of androgen therapy for females that use the natural hormone, which reduces potential side effects. A testosterone patch has been used in men, and is being developed for use by women.

For women, one or two 75 mg pellets of testosterone may be implanted subcutaneously (these last four to six months) with the estrogen replacement given orally, by one or two implanted Estradiol pellets 25 mg, or by transdermal (estradiol) patch. Oral progestogens should also be added from the 13th to the 25th of the month.

Testosterone gel can be obtained from a compounding pharmacist and used daily. The dosage of testosterone gel should be limited to 10–20% of the gel available for men, or 5 to 10 mg testosterone per 5 gm of gel.

TABLE 16.1: ANDROGENS

Name	Androgen	mg/Ml	Manufacturer
Oral Androgens			
Generic	methyltestosterone	5mg	
Generic	fluoxymesterone	2mg	
		5mg	
Injectables			
Depo-testosterone	testosterone cypionate	100mg/ml 200mg/ml	Pharmacia
Delatestryl	testosterone enanthate	100mg/ml	Squibb
Testopel	testosterone pellets	75mg/ml	
Estrogen/Androgen Combinations			
Estratest tablets	esterified estrogens methyltestosterone	1.25mg 2.50mg	Solvay
Estratest H.S. tablets	esterified estrogens methyltestosterone	0.625mg 1.25mg	Solvay
Depo Testadiol	estradiol cypionate Testosterone cypionate	2mg 50mg	
Estradiol USP*	estradiol pellet (given with testosterone pellets)	25mg	Various Pharmacies

* Available from certain pharmacies

NOTES

#	Topic	Section
1.	Introduction	Indications
2.	Vasomoter Symptoms	
3.	Urogenital Atrophy	
4.	Psychogenic Manifestations	
5.	Osteoporosis	
6.	Coronary Artery Disease (CAD)	
7.	Alzheimer's Disease (AD)	
8.	The Women's Health Initiative (WHI)	
9.	Vaginal Hormonal Cytology	Evaluation
10.	Progestogen Challenge Test	
11.	Endometrial Biopsy	
12.	Osteoporosis Detection Methods	
13.	Laboratory and Tests for Early Cancer Detection	
14.	Oral Estrogens	Hormone Replacement
15.	Non-Oral Estrogens	
16.	Androgens	

Hormone Replacement (continued)	Progestogens	17.
	Selective Estrogen Receptor Modulators (SERMS)	18.
	Oral Contraceptives	19.
Calcium	Calcium Supplements	20.
Risks	Endometrial Hyperplasia	21.
	Endometrial Cancer	22.
	Hormones and Breast Cancer	23.
	Thromboembolic Disease	24.
	Hypertension	25.
	Gallbladder Disease	26.
	Nutrition and Diet	27.
	Lipid Metabolism	28.
Side Effects	Management of Side Effects	29.
	Contraindications	30.
	Alternative Therapy	31.
References	References/Manufacturer's Listing	32.

SECTION 17: PROGESTOGENS

Clinical Information
There are three ways that progestogens are commonly used in estrogen replacement therapy. These are:
- Annually, in the progestogen challenge test
- Cyclically, to oppose estrogen effects
- Continuously, to oppose estrogen and induce amenorrhea

Progestogen Challenge Test
The progestogen challenge test should be performed on all climacteric women who have intact uteri and who are:
- Asymptomatic and have regular annual examination
- Symptomatic and are being evaluated for estrogen therapy
- Currently on unopposed estrogen therapy

In the testing procedure, the patient takes 13 days of progestogen (see Table 17.1). If withdrawal bleeding occurs, progestogens should be added to the estrogen therapy from the 13th to the 25th of each monthly cycle. If there is no response, the progestogen challenge test should be repeated annually for asymptomatic women who are not using hormones.

Cyclic Use of Progestogens
Progestogens are increasingly being added to estrogen replacement therapy for postmenopausal women. In the 1970s, studies revealed that unopposed estrogen replacement therapy increases the risk of endometrial cancer. Therefore, reasons for adding progestogens to estrogen replacement include:
- Prevention of endometrial cancer
- Reduction in risk of breast cancer
- Promotion of new bone formation
- Prevention and treatment of osteoporosis

Some troublesome effects of unopposed estrogen (e.g., breast tenderness) may be alleviated by adding progestogens. Although added progestogen may aggravate mastodynia when initiating therapy, this usually abates with time. Edema, bloating, and irritability are more frequent in women taking unopposed estrogens but are sometimes aggravated by added progestogen.

Other uses of progestogens during the climacteric include:
- Preventing vasomotor flushes
- Avoiding annual endometrial biopsies
- Decreasing the frequency of biopsies performed for abnormal postmenopausal bleeding

One major drawback is that the same contraindications are listed for progestogens as for estrogens. However, this labeling should not preclude physicians from using their best judgment in the interest of their patients.

There is no good evidence that progestogens have an adverse reaction on coagulation factors or mammary tissue in humans.

There are also concerns about the long-term effects of progestogens, particularly with possible adverse effects on HDL cholesterol (see Section 28). Some patients are reluctant to resume menstruation and sometimes experience premenstrual-like symptoms during progestogen therapy. However, after menopause, menstrual effects are lessened for patients taking progestogens, including:
- Reduced menstrual flow (three to four days)
- Lessened dysmenorrhea
- Lessened PMS

Research has demonstrated a reduction in abnormal postmenopausal bleeding. In one study, abnormal bleeding occurred in 23.3 percent of non-users of hormones, 14.2 percent of users of estrogen alone, and in only 3.9 percent of estrogen-progestogen users {51}.

Although any unscheduled bleeding should be promptly investigated, annual endometrial biopsies are not required for users of progestogens. One study showed that hyperplasia or neoplasia occurred in 8.1 percent of non-users, 7.9 percent of estrogen users, and 0.9 percent of estrogen-progestogen users.

Adding Progestogen to Estrogen Replacement

Patients with intact uterus receiving oral estrogens from the first through the 25th of each month should have the progestogen added (see Table 17.1) from the 13th through the 25th for the benefit of the bones and the breasts (see Sections 5 and 23). Women who have had hysterectomy only need the progestogen for the first 10 days each month to reduce their risk of breast cancer. They also can use lower dosages such as norethindrone acetate 2.5 mg or Prometrium 100 mg.

Women on continuous estrogen, injectables, or estradiol pellet implants may be given the progestogen the first 13 days of each month.

For initial therapy, C-21 progestogens (e.g., medroxyprogesterone acetate 10 mg) should be chosen for women with histories of breast problems such as fibrocystic disease or mastodynia. The 19-nor-steroid progestogens (e.g., norethindrone acetate 2.5 or 5 mg) are best for those with histories of heavy or prolonged menstrual periods.

Studies show that less than 10 mg of Provera may not be protective for the endometrium {44}. Although 5 mg of norethindrone acetate is the recommended starting dosage, as little as 1 mg of norethindrone may be protective for the endometrium. Therefore, the trend is toward lower dosage of the 19-nor-steroid progestogens (e.g., 2.5 mg of norethindrone acetate).

Injectable progestogens are not recommended for postmenopausal women with intact uteri, since the duration of action is irregular and breakthrough bleeding may result.

Continuous combined estrogen-progesterone therapy is available in several combinations. They can be used for patients who do not want withdrawal bleeding. We recommend using it for 25 days each month to prevent endometrial hyperplasia as it gives the chance for the estradiol and progesterone receptors to regenerate. If there is any abnormal bleeding on this therapy endometrial sampling is advised.

Side Effects of Estrogen-Progestogen Therapy

The major side effect of estrogen-progestogen therapy is that 97 percent of patients have withdrawal bleeding until age 60, with 60 percent of patients continuing withdrawal bleeding after age 65. In addition, five to 10 percent of patients experience:
- Breast tenderness
- Edema
- Bloating
- Premenstrual irritability
- Lower abdominal cramps
- Dysmenorrhea

Patient acceptance of withdrawal bleeding has been good once the benefits are clearly explained. However, patients do not have to accept continued menses with alternative methods of combination estrogen-progestogen therapy.

Side effects may be managed by:
- Decreasing the estrogen dosage
- Adding a mild diuretic:
  - HCTZ, 25 to 50 mg, OR
  - Spironolactone, 25 to 50 mg
- Changing to another progestogen

For patients who cannot tolerate any oral progestogen, progesterone suppositories (50 mg daily) may be used in divided dosages {47}. Also, oral micronized progesterone is available from certain pharmacies and is now commercially available as *Prometrium*. The dosage is 300 mm daily in divided dosages, 100 mg in the morning and 200 mg at bedtime, since the major side effect is drowsiness.

General aches and pains can be dealt with by using a prostaglandin-inhibiting analgesic such as:
- Aspirin
- Ibuprofen, 400 to 800 mg four times daily

- Naproxen, 250 to 500 mg three times daily
- Naproxen Sodium, 275 to 550 mg three times daily (*Aleve*, 220 mg)

These NSAIDs are excellent for menstrual cramps since they inhibit prostaglandin synthesis, one cause of dysmenorrhea.

TABLE 17.1: PROGESTOGENS

	Brand Name	Manufacturer	Available Dosage Forms	Usual Maintenance Dose
Medroxyprogesterone acetate		Watson	2.5mg,5mg,10mg tablet	5–10mg PO qd for 12–14d
Norethindrone	Nor-QD	Watson	0.35mg tablet	—
Norethindrone	Micronor	Ortho-McNeil	0.35mg tablet	0.7mg PO qd for 12–14d
Norethindrone acetate			5mg tablet	5mg PO qd for 12–14d
Norgestrel	Ovrette	Wyeth	0.075mg tablet	0.15mg PO qd for 12–14d
Progesterone	Prometrium	Solvay	100mg,200mg capsule	100 in am and 200mg hs 12–14d

SECTION 18: SELECTIVE ESTROGEN RECEPTOR MODULATORS (SERMS)

The approval of the selective estrogen receptor modulators (SERMS) such as raloxifene, *(Evista)* and tamoxifen has given a new dimension to the treatment of menopause. Unfortunately, many patients develop severe hot flashes due to the anti-estrogen effect. There are patients who do not desire estrogen replacement based on fear generated from media articles. There are also those who do not desire to continue hormone therapy for a prolonged period of time, but may benefit from raloxifene therapy.

The SERMS have estrogen-like action on the bone and anti-estrogen effects on the endometrium and breast. Tamoxifen has shown benefits in protecting against breast cancer, and preserving bone and cardiovascular health, but seems to increase endometrial cancer risk. The newer SERM raloxifene seems to have similar effects, but does not seem to have the stimulatory effect on the endometrium.

Raloxifene and Cardiovascular Disease

In the Multiple Outcomes of Raloxifene Evaluation (MORE), there was no increased risk for the coronary or cerebrovascular events at the 60 mg or 120 mg dose compared to placebo {41}. Raloxifene Use for The Heart (RUTH) is the new study being conducted world wide to evaluate cardiovascular benefit.

Osteoporosis:

A dosage of 60 mg of raloxifene is approved for both prevention and treatment of osteoporosis. Vertebral fractures were decreased by 55% in patients without pre-existing fractures, and by 30% in patients with fractures. There was no benefit on the hip fracture incidence, but there was increase in bone mineral density.

Breast Cancer:

Raloxifene seems to reduce the incidence of breast cancer and studies are being done to evaluate the same.

Vasomotor Symptoms:

Hot flashes seem to be increased in younger post-menopausal patients, but may not be so severe in the older menopausal female.

Thromboembolism:

The incidence of increase in thrombotic events was similar to estrogen replacement.

Raloxifene is a good alternative for patients who do not want to take hormone therapy to protect against osteoporosis, and could have all the benefits of estrogen, such as reducing the risk of AD and prevention of macular degeneration of the retina, but this has not been proven.

SECTION 19: ORAL CONTRACEPTIVES

There are greater doses of estrogen and progestogen in oral contraceptives than are needed to treat postmenopausal women. Even the lowest dose oral contraceptive has 20 µg of ethinyl estradiol and 1 mg of norethindrone acetate. Five µg of ethinyl estradiol, particularly when combined with a progestogen, will prevent osteoporosis and relieve menopausal symptoms. However, with the increasing recognition of side benefits, rather than negative side effects, birth control pills should be encouraged for perimenopausal nonsmokers needing family planning. Smokers ages 40 and older should be encouraged to stop smoking so that they can also reap these benefits.

Non-contraceptive Health Benefits

Noncontraceptive health benefits of oral contraceptives are:
- Decreased risks of:
  - Endometrial cancer
  - Ovarian cancer
  - Ovarian cysts
- Less benign breast disease
- Probably less breast cancer
- Treatment of:
  - Dysfunctional uterine bleeding
  - Dysmenorrhea
  - Hirsutism
  - Acne
  - Endometriosis
- Decreased:
  - Iron deficiency anemia
  - Thyroid disease
- Less rheumatoid arthritis
- Effective contraception
- Decreased:
  - Ectopic pregnancy
  - Pelvic inflammatory disease
- Increased bone mass

Breast Cancer

Although this remains controversial, there is no evidence from the more than 100 studies that oral contraceptive use increases the risk of carcinoma of the breast {26,138}. In fact, the contrary could be true. In one of the largest studies of women whose carcinoma of the breast was diagnosed between ages 45 and 54, those who had used birth control pills had a slightly decreased risk of breast cancer (RR = 0.9; 95% CI, 0.8 to 1.0) {174}. Among these women, the risk estimates decreased significantly ($P \leq 0.01$) with increasing time between first and last use.

Not only do oral contraceptives significantly reduce the risk of benign breast disease, but birth control pills and progestogens reverse both intraductal hyperplasia and atypia of the breast, which may be precancerous lesions {169}.

SECTION 20: CALCIUM SUPPLEMENTS

Clinical Information

Bone loss due to osteoporosis is associated with alterations in calcium metabolism yielding negative calcium balance. Although calcium intake does not decrease at the time of menopause and calcium absorption does not vary greatly, a rise in fasting urinary calcium is found at about this time {117}.

As determined by the NIH Consensus Conference on Osteoporosis, the American diet is deficient in calcium intake, particularly among women who diet to maintain a thin figure {115}. The usual daily intake of elemental calcium in the United States, 450 to 550 mg, is below the National Research Council's recommended dietary allowance (RDA) of 800 mg per day. Calcium metabolic balance studies indicate a daily requirement of 1,000 mg of elemental calcium for premenopausal and estrogen-treated postmenopausal women. Postmenopausal women who are not treated with estrogens require 1,500 mg or more daily for calcium balance.

Calcium Level Changes

Changes in urinary calcium levels are difficult to detect since 24-hour collections reflect absorbed dietary calcium. Patients must be studied in a fasting state when urinary calcium derives primarily from bone.

By comparing fasting calcium levels in hysterectomized women who also had bilateral oophorectomy to those who had ovarian conservation, the increase in resorption of calcium from bone can be related to reduced ovarian estrogens {117}. Both fasting plasma and urinary hydroxyproline confirm that the increased calcium excretion is due to increased bone resorption of calcium. Women undergoing natural menopause have similar changes in calcium metabolism. Postmenopausal women show a higher morning fasting urinary calcium-to-creatinine ratio than premenopausal women.

The increase in fasting serum or urinary calcium that follows either natural menopause or bilateral oophorectomy is reversible with estrogen therapy. Estrogen administration also stimulates calcitonin production, which is decreased after menopause, and may affect bone calcium indirectly since calcitonin is known to inhibit bone resorption. Adding progestogen to estrogen replacement therapy enhances the effects of the estrogen, thereby promoting new bone formation {122}.

Recommendations

As recommended by the NIH Consensus Conference on Osteoporosis, calcium supplements are essential but of secondary importance to estrogen replacement. Weight-bearing exercise was the third recommendation. A few studies have shown a reduction in fracture rate with calcium alone. However, most studies have also used estrogen replacement plus calcium.

Calcium carbonate is the most widely-studied calcium and probably the best absorbed, with 40 percent absorbed as elemental calcium. Other calcium products can be used, but amounts absorbed as elemental calcium vary. For example, only 10 percent of calcium lactate is absorbed as calcium. Most of the calcium makers now list the amount of elemental calcium in their products rather than the total mg of calcium in each tablet (see Table 20.1).

Calcium supplementation should be started by age 35 to 40. This is when women have peak bone mass. Women whose diets are markedly deficient in calcium should start supplementation earlier {117}. The more bone mass a women has entering menopause, the more she is apt to retain.

The major sources of calcium in the United States diet are milk and dairy products. Each eight ounce glass of milk contains 275 to 300 mg of calcium. Skim milk may actually contain more calcium. Other dietary sources of calcium include:
- Low fat yogurt
- Cheese

- Fish, particularly those canned with bones
- Clams, oysters, and shrimp
- Spinach, broccoli, leafy vegetables
- Peanuts, almonds, brazil nuts
- Tofu
- Calcium-fortified orange juice

Other agents that may be helpful in preventing osteoporosis include (92}:
- Vitamin D or analogues
- Sodium fluoride
- Calcitriol
- Calcitonin
- Anabolic steroids
- Thiazide diuretics
- Magnesium
- Etidronate
- Alendronate
- Residronate
- Raloxifene
- PTH injectable
- Miacalcin Nasal Spray

More research needs to be done with these agents before they can be widely recommended. Calcitonin (*Calcimar*—USV Laboratories) at 100 IU daily by injection (subcutaneous or IM) is probably the best substitute for estrogen replacement when estrogens are contraindicated. Injectible parathyroid hormone (PTH) is very promising.

Intranasal calcitonin (*Miacalcin*—Sandoz) has been approved for use in the U.S. An intranasal daily dose of 200 IU was able to maintain bone mass in both the spine and femur {55,117}. Calcitonin seems to be more effective in the period more than five years after menopause, but not as effective as estrogen and the bisphosphonates.

TABLE 20.1: CALCIUM SUPPLEMENTS

Name	Calcium	Elemental Ca	Manufacturer
Os-Cal 500	calcium carbonate	500 mg	Marion
Os-Cal 250	calcium carbonate + Vit D	250 mg	Marion
Posture	calcium phosphate	600 mg	Whitehall
Posture with D	calcium phosphate + Vit D	600 mg	Whitehall
Caltrate 600	calcium carbonate	600 mg	Lederle
Caltrate 600 + Vit D	calcium carbonate + Vit D	600 mg	Lederle
Citracal	calcium citrate	200 mg	Mission
Calcet	calcium lactate	152.8 mg	Mission
	calcium gluconate		
	calcium carbonate		
Nutravescent	calcium citrate + V + D	500 mg	Northhampton
Tums	calcium carbonate	200 mg	Smithkline Beecham
Tums-EX	calcium carbonate	300 mg	
Tums 500	calcium carbonate	500 mg	
Viactive (chewable)	calcium carbonate	500 mg	Merck

SECTION 21: ENDOMETRIAL HYPERPLASIA

Research

Hyperplasia of the endometrium has been established as a pre-cancerous lesion in some women. In a prospective study of 562 women with adenomatous hyperplasia, 18.5 percent developed cancer after a few years. By the tenth year, the incidence of adenocarcinoma rose to 30 percent {63}.

In another study, 115 patients with hyperplasia or adenocarcinoma *in situ* were followed for two to eight years without any therapy, either hysterectomy or hormonal manipulation. A significant number developed invasive adenocarcinoma {170}, including:

- 26.7 percent of those with adenomatous hyperplasia
- 81.8 percent of those with atypical hyperplasia
- 100 percent of those with adenocarcinoma *in situ*

Of the 31 patients with endometrial cancer in the Wilford Hall USAF Medical Center study, 11 (39.3 percent) had a previous diagnosis of hyperplasia from four months to eight years before detection of cancer {46}. Although earlier studies contend that adenomatous hyperplasia may be pre-cancerous, any degree of hyperplasia may be significant since six of these 11 patients had only benign or cystic hyperplasia, yet developed endometrial cancer in a relatively short period of time.

In a five-year prospective study, 325 women were found to have varying degrees of endometrial hyperplasia {45}. They were treated with progestogens for seven to 10 days each month for three to six months and curettage was repeated after therapy. Hyperplasia reversed to normal endometrium in 307 (94.5 percent). Of the 18 patients with persistent hyperplasia, 14 had been given progestogens for only seven days each month; only four patients with persistent hyperplasia had been treated for 10 days monthly (see Table 21.1).

For the past 25 years in our practice endometrial hyperplasia has been successfully reversed to a normal endometrium within six months by using progestogens 13 days monthly (see Table 21.2).

Hyperplasia and Estrogen Replacement Therapy

Unopposed estrogens have a role in the development of endometrial hyperplasia and neoplasia, primarily because of incomplete shedding of the endometrium. Progesterone or progestogen therapy ensures more complete sloughing of the endometrium, leaving behind fewer glands and cells for continued proliferation and growth. The protective action of progestogens on the endometrium is primarily physical. However, additional actions of both natural progesterone and synthetic progestogens may be important. Progestogens decrease estrogen receptors in endometrial cells and induce estradiol dehydrogenase and isocitrate activity, which are the mechanisms by whose means these cells metabolize estrogens.

Recommendations for Treatment

The preferred method of treatment of endometrial hyperplasia is an initial curettage followed by a course of progestogen therapy (see Table 17.1). Norethindrone acetate 5 mg, or medroxyprogesterone acetate 10 mg, should be taken for 13 days monthly. After six months of progestogen therapy, the curettage should be repeated. If the endometrial hyperplasia is persistent, hysterectomy is recommended.

If the patient is on estrogen therapy, discontinuance is not necessary during the six months of progestogen therapy. The hyperplasia will reverse equally well on combined estrogen-progestogen therapy.

TABLE 21.1: EFFECTS OF PROGESTOGENS ON ENDOMETRIAL HYPERPLASIA
(Total number of patients: 325)

Pathology Before Therapy	Number of Patients
Benign hyperplasia	196
Cystic hyperplasia	34
Adenomatous hyperplasia	28
A-typical adenomatous hyperplasia	67
Endometrium After Therapy	**Number of Patients**
Proliferative	156
Secretory	69
Atrophic	53
Dyssynchronous maturation	29
Benign hyperplasia	12
Adenomatous hyperplasia	4
A-typical adenomatous hyperplasia	2

Incidence of endometrial cancer in the various treatment groups compared with untreated from 1975–1983
(Reproduced with permission from Gambrell) {46}.

TABLE 21.2: REVERSAL OF HYPERPLASIA WITH INCREASED DURATION OF PROGESTOGENS

Number Of Patients with Hyperplasia	Duration of Progestogens (Days)	Persistent Hyperplasia	% Reversal
72	7	14	80.6
253	10	4	98.4
45	13	0	100.0

SECTION 22: ENDOMETRIAL CANCER

Clinical Information

Unopposed estrogen therapy increases the risk of endometrial cancer, although the magnitude has been exaggerated by the methodology used in retrospective studies {93,141,144,178}. Progestogen added to estrogen replacement therapy for 12 to 14 days per month reduces the risk of endometrial adenocarcinoma to less than that of untreated women {44,46,49,65,112}. For those not needing estrogen replacement, use of the progestogen challenge test to screen asymptomatic postmenopausal women can reduce adenocarcinoma of the endometrium {46,49}.

Not all postmenopausal women need estrogen. Many produce sufficient endogenous estrogens to remain asymptomatic and prevent the metabolic changes of long-term estrogen deficiency in later life. However, within this group may be those in need of progestogen to prevent endometrial hyperplasia, possibly leading to endometrial carcinoma. The progestogen challenge test (see Section 10) was devised to identify those in this high-risk group. A positive response to this test (withdrawal bleeding) indicates that 13 days per month of progestogen therapy should be continued for as long as withdrawal bleeding occurs in order to ensure complete endometrial shedding.

Research

During the five years of prospective study and four years of follow-up at Wilford Hall USAF Medical Center from 1975 to 1983 (Figure 22.1), 5,563 post-menopausal women were registered in the hormone user survey {46}. However, approximately 40 percent had hysterectomies and were not at risk for endometrial cancer. Adenocarcinoma of the endometrium was diagnosed in 31 patients during 27,243 patient-years of observation, for an overall incidence of 113.8 per 100,000 women per year (see Table 22.1).

The largest group of patients, the estrogen-progestogen users, with 16,327 patient-years of observation, was found to have eight cancers for an annual incidence of 49.0 per 100,000 women. The highest incidence of endometrial carcinoma was observed in the unopposed estrogen users, in whom 10 cancers were detected during 2,560 patient-years, for an incidence of 390.6 per 100,000 women. The second highest incidence was 11 cancers in the non-users of hormones during 4,480 patient-years of observation, for an incidence of 245.5 per 100,000 women. Only two endometrial cancers were observed in the estrogen vaginal cream users, and no malignancies occurred in either the progestogen or androgen users. This group consisted primarily of progestogen users, women who had been identified as being at increased risk for adenocarcinoma by the progestogen challenge test and who were being treated with cyclic progestogens only.

Other studies have demonstrated the efficacy of progestogens in protecting estrogen users from adenocarcinoma. One reported no endometrial cancers in 72 estrogen-progestogen users, but 11 cancers in 207 patients treated with unopposed estrogens {65}. In a double-blind study, no adenocarcinomas were diagnosed in the 84 patients using estrogen-progestogen for 10 years, but one endometrial cancer occurred in the 84 placebo users {103}. Studies from England have not uncovered any increased risk for endometrial malignancy in estrogen-treated postmenopausal women, because they routinely add a progestogen {160}. However, a 15-percent endometrial hyperplasia rate was observed in the unopposed estrogen users before progestogens were added {160}.

The increasing addition of progestogens to estrogen replacement therapy is already having a beneficial effect on the national incidence of endometrial cancer. Figure 22.2 compares the 1973 to 1987 SEER incidence of endometrial cancer by age when mostly unopposed estrogen was used {105} to the 1981 to 1985 SEER incidence when progestogens were being increasingly added to estrogen replacement {4}. The trend shown is a shift downward in incidence and to a later age, confirming the effectiveness of adding progestogens.

Cases of Endometrial Cancer with Estrogen-Progestogen Use

In a current review, there were 66 cases of endometrial cancer reported with estrogen-progestogen use {49}. The vast majority occurred when too low a dosage of progestogen, or too short a duration of progestogen, was given. There are no cases of endometrial cancer reported when 10 mg of medroxyprogesterone acetate or 5 mg of norethindrone acetate was prescribed for 12 to 14 days each month.

The continuous combined method of hormone replacement may not be fully endometrial-protective, since 15 of the reported cases of cancer were using this regimen {27,38,52,56,87}. In addition to these 15 reported cases, the author has learned of 123 additional cases of endometrial cancer, including two deaths, for a total of 138; this may only be the tip of the iceberg. Since these cases did not begin to appear until a decade of ever increasing usage of the continuous combined hormone replacement regimen and most occurred after two to four years of amenorrhea, the one to three years' published studies were of insufficient duration to demonstrate safety. It may be very important to withdraw the progestogen for a few days each month to allow any build-up of endometrium to be shed. This is the way that the normal ovulatory cycle, sequential estrogen-progestogen therapy, and oral contraceptives work to decrease the risk of endometrial cancer. Ultrasonography can be performed to evaluate the endometrial thickness, and if it is greater than 5 mm endometrial biopsy is recommended. Also, any abnormal bleeding should be evaluated by endometrial sampling.

A Better Method?

For the past fifteen years, the author has used the cyclic combined regimen to produce amenorrhea {32}. Low dosage estrogen and progestogen (2.5 mg of medroxyprogesterone acetate or 2.5 mg of norethindrone acetate) are given by the calendar from the first through the 25th of each month.

This is clinically superior to the continuous combined method in that after comparable spotting during the first month of therapy, there is less breakthrough bleeding, usually one or two days of spotting on the 26th or 27th. More women will become amenorrheic by four months (75 percent) compared to 60 to 65 percent with the continuous combined regimen.

When bleeding does occur with the cyclic combined method, it is usually only one or two days of spotting on the 26th or 27th, which most women can accept when full explanation and reassurance are given.

The cyclic combined regimen should be more endometrial-protective than the continuous combined method since we now have fifteen years of experience. Theoretically, the regimen should be protective, since discontinuing the progestogen should allow for shedding any build-up of endometrium.

Another promising method of HRT that is endometrial-protective, and also produces more amenorrhea than continuous combined HRT, is interrupted progestogen, or pulsed progestogen {14,16,155}. Available as a combination patch in England, estradial 0.5 mg only is applied for four days followed by estradiol 0.5 mg, plus 0.250 mg norethindrone acetate for three days {14}. Relief of hot flashes and amenorrhea was achieved in 71 percent by six months. An oral interrupted progestogen combined with micronized estradiol 1 mg is available in the United States as *Prefest* {155}. The estrogen alone for three days, then combined with norgestimate 0.09 mg for three days, produced amenorrhea in 80 percent by one year. The three to four days without progestogen allows upregulation of progesterone receptors in the endometrium {16}. Continuous down regulation of progesterone receptor with continuous combined HRT is a major reason this method is not fully endometrial-protective.

TABLE 22.1: INCIDENCE OF ENDOMETRIAL CANCER AT WILFORD HALL USAF MEDICAL CENTER: 1975–1983

Therapy Group	Patient-Years of Ovservation	Patients with Cancer	Incidence (Per 100,000)
Estroge-Progestogen Users	16,327	8	49.0
Unopposed Estrogen Users	2,560	10	390.6
Estrogen Vaginal Cream Users	2,716	2	73.6
Progestogen Users	1,160	0	x
Non-Users	4,480	11	245.5
TOTAL	27,243	31	113.8

FIGURE 22.1—Incidence Of Endometrial Cancer

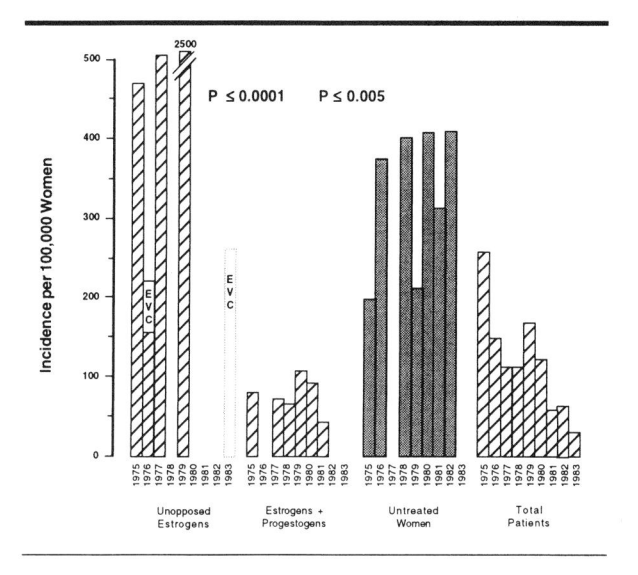

Incidence of endometrial cancer in the various treatment groups compared with untreated from 1975–1983. {46}

FIGURE 22.2—Changing Incidence of Endometrial Cancer

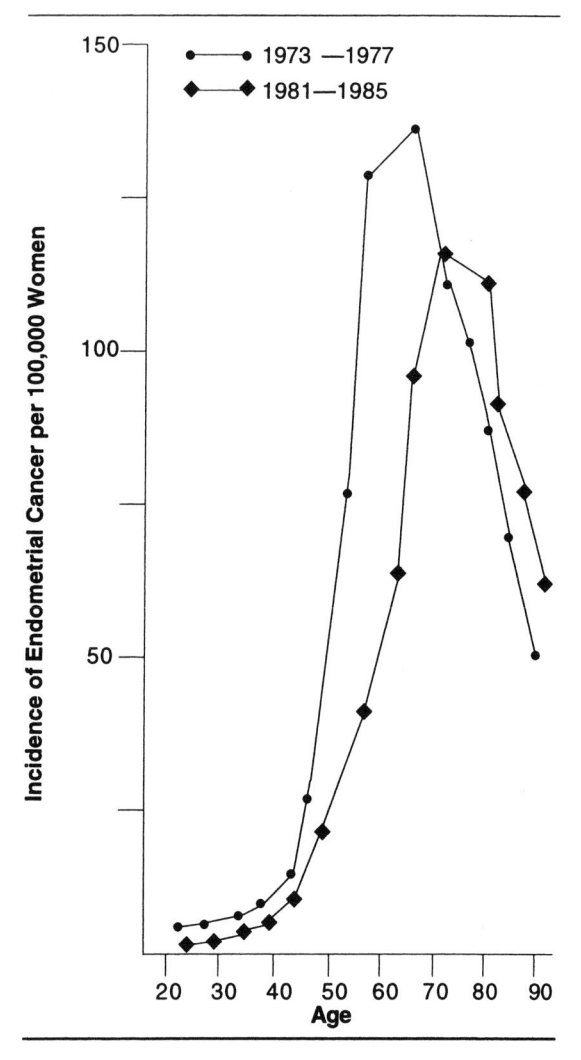

The shifting of endometrial cancer in women by age between 1973–1977 and 1981–1985.

NOTES

SECTION 23: HORMONES AND BREAST CANCER

Clinical Information

One of the greatest concerns women have is the development of breast cancer during their life time. Breast cancer is being diagnosed in early stages due to increasing utilization of mammograms (up to 60% in women over age 50) and greater public awareness of the disease. It is the most common malignancy in the United States comprising 32% of all female cancers and 15% of all cancer deaths, second only to lung cancer {59,79}. Mortality from breast cancer is on the decline from 46,000 in 1995 to 40,110 deaths in 2004. Incidence of breast cancer world wide is 35.6 per 100,000 females. Deaths from breast cancer in the United States is 21.2 per 100,000 women, which ranks 12th in the world. The leader is Denmark with 29.2 deaths per 100,000. China has the lowest mortality at 4.5 per 100,000 {80}.

Risk Factors

There have been several factors implicated in the development of breast cancer. Age (Figure 23.1) and family history are the most prominent. Other factors include:

a) Excessive alcohol intake—Women who drink two to five drinks a day run a 41% greater risk of developing breast cancer than non-drinkers {17}

b) Obesity—Post menopausal women who gain 11 to 22 pounds have an 18% higher risk of breast cancer than women who gain four to five pounds. In those who gain 44 to 55 pounds the risk jumps to 40% {161}. It has been suggested that eating a diet rich in soy products, olive oil, oils rich in non-saturated fats, and green leafy vegetables may decrease risk of developing breast cancer {71}.

c) Genetic factors—Female relatives of women with breast cancer have a higher risk when compared to general population {135}. The risks are as follows:

- Affected mother *or* sister   2 to 3 RR
- Aunt or grandmother   1.5 RR
- Affected mother *and* sister   14.0 RR

d) Estrogens—The role, mechanism and molecular factors: The most controversial among the risk factors has been the association of estrogens with breast cancer. Experimental data have shown that estrogens may play a role in the development of breast cancer in some women. Alkylation of cellular molecule and generation of active radicals can damage the DNA in association with potential genotoxicity of estrogen metabolites, namely catechol estrogens. This may be due to the direct effect of the enzymes and proteins by stimulating prolactin and growth factors {176}. Indirect evidence of this includes increased rate of breast cancer associated with early menarche, delayed pregnancy, late menopause and decreased rate in women who develop early menopause {128}. Obese postmenopausal women have higher concentrations of bio active estrogens and it is well known that obesity increases the risk {161}.

Association of role of exogenous estrogens is controversial at best. There is no evidence of increased risk in women using oral contraceptives {26,66}. There have been some subgroups among women who start birth control at an early age; those that take it for a long time, or those currently using it, may have an increased risk {168}. Risk is not increased in those who have discontinued birth control for more than 10 years.

Estrogen therapy (ET) and hormone therapy (EPT) have been implicated as a risk factor for many years and the increase seems to be related to the duration of use {25,94,137}. The overall mortality in ERT users has been lower than non-users {48,60}. Family history of breast cancer is not modified by the use of birth control pills or after ET/EPT, but some feel use of estrogen may increase the risk in breast cancer genes (BrCa 1 and BrCa 2) {21,24,166}.

ET, EPT, and the recent Breast Cancer Controversy

The report of the Women's Heatlh Initiative (WHI) sponsored by National Institutes of Health (NIH) has raised much concern regarding the role of hormones and breast cancer {131}. This has caused widespread discontinuation of the hormones and deprives the women of the benefit of hormones. The study was discontinued prematurely at 5.2 years of follow-up, vs the planned 8.5 years. This is too short an interval. Even the 8.5 years is not long enough as it takes more than 8 years for the discovery of breast cancer from a single cell based on doubling times. Based on this all of the 290 cases of breast cancer had malignant cells at the onset of the study. The trial of EPT with continuous combined estrogen-progestin was stopped due to minimal increase of hazard ratio (HR) of 1.26, which was only of borderline significance, 1.00-1.59, which is not clinically relevant. The study of estrogen alone has not shown an increase in the risk of breast cancer at 7 years {159}. It will take at least 15 years to reveal the actual risks. In the HERS study, which also included the continuous combined HRT, the increase was RR = 1.27 (95% CI, 0.84–1.94), which was not significant {76}.

Do Exogenous Estrogens Cause Cancer? Role of Progestogens

There is confirming evidence from more than seventy studies that exogenous therapy, and even unopposed estrogens, do not increase the risk for breast cancer {12,23,24,48}. There have been eleven studies, with none to the contrary, that have examined survival from breast cancer developing in estrogen users and have observed lower mortality {12,24,45,48,60,68,78,107,136,151,172}. Long term progesterone deficiency has been shown to increase the risk of breast cancer {28,29,98,126}. Megesterol acetate and medroxyprogesterone acetate have been equally effective to tamoxifen in reducing recurrences of breast cancer {13}. In one study, in patients with stage IV metastatic breast cancer, estrogen with high dose progestogen was shown to be very effective {75}. After giving estrogens for seven days to enhance the progesterone receptors in metastatic cancer cells high dose medroxyprogesterone acetate was given and the remission rate was 56% for up to six years. Oral contraceptives and progestogens seem to reverse intraductal hyperplasia and atypia of breast {169}. In a study of 1150 menopausal women with benign breast disease, treatment with progestins for more than 10 years significantly decreased the risk of breast cancer {120}.

The most consistently decreased risk of breast cancer in estrogen users has been those who also received progestogens. Four of the eight studies found a decrease compared to placebo treated controls or never-users {46,86,104,149}. The Danish and Swedish studies, and the study from the National Cancer Institute (NCI) found a non-significantly increased risk of mammary cancer in estrogen-progestogen users {42,118,137}. The Danish study was only a five year study, and the Swedish study was based on 16 patients and ten years of use. In the NCI study only 4% of the 2082 breast cancer patients were estrogen-progestogen users. This risk went away four to six years after discontinuation. In a study from southern California estrogen alone did not increase the risk; nor did continuous combined EPT {130}. The Seattle study observed a 60% decrease (RR = 0.4) in cancer risk with eight or more years of estrogen –progesterone use {149}. In the Wilford Hall studies the lowest incidence of breast cancer was in the estrogen-progestogen users at 66.8 per 100,000 women per year (see Table 23.1) {46}. The incidence in the unopposed estrogen users was 142.3 per 100,000 and in the non-users it was 342.3 per 100,000 women per year. As progestogen was increasingly added to estrogen therapy the incidence of breast cancer steadily declined (see Figure 23.2 and Figure 23.3). Nachtigall's study followed the patients for 22 years on estrogen plus progestogen, and Lauritzen followed the patients for 20 years; both of them found a decrease in the risk of breast cancer {86,104}. In the longest prospective study to date there were no breast cancers during the 22 years in the 116 estrogen-progestogen users while six cases developed breast cancer {104}.

The Nurses Health Study is the only study to show an increase in breast cancer—RR 1.32 {23}. The Iowa study revealed a better histology and found no increased risk in the hormone group {54}. In another study there was an elevated risk of lobular carcinoma, but no increase in ductal cancer {89}.

Recently Bush and colleagues compared the age adjusted risk estimates for breast cancer among ever-users of estrogen therapy compared with non-users from 45 previously published articles that assessed ERT and breast cancer risk, and 20 articles that assessed HRT and breast cancer risk {12}. In addition 11 studies were assessed for risk estimates for death from breast cancer and breast cancer survival. They found little consistency in the studies that estimated the risk of breast cancer in the hormone users, versus the non-users, but there was consistenly lower mortality in the users than non-users. Most of the studies reported a relative risk of 0.9 to 1 for development of breast cancer. None of the studies had increased risk, while two found protective effect and one no increased risk. The risk estimates for deaths from breast cancer was consistently less in hormone users compared to non-users. Others have also shown that estrogen users are less likely to die than non-users after a breast cancer diagnosis {60,151,172}.

Can We Use Estrogens After Breast Cancer?

Most physicians believe once a patient has breast cancer estrogens should not be used. However, several recent studies have shown that estrogens can be used safely in properly selected patients, after a thorough discussion with the patients about the benefits and risks.

It is well known that premenopausal women who develop beast cancer continue to produce estrogens, but they are denied the hormones when they reach menopause {30}. Five year survival has increased from 72% to 97% in recent years {59}. There have been several studies that have addressed the use of ERT/HRT after early breast cancer to treat menopausal symptoms and protect against osteoporosis {20,21,34,35,36,37,40,106,107,111,121,150,165,167,171}.

In our first report we had 75 patients with early breast cancer. Fifty received estrogens and mortality was significantly lower in the estrogen group {106}. In our subsequent study there were 123 patients ranging in age from 39 to 91 years; 69 patients received ERT/EPT for up to 32 years. Twenty-two received non-hormonal therapy, and 32 who received no treatment {107}. Mortality rate in the estrogen group was 4.28% compared to 11.3% in non-users {107}. O'Meara and colleagues compiled data from 2,755 women aged 35 to 74 years to evaluate the impact of ERT/HRT on breast cancer survival and recurrence {111}. There were 174 patients who received HRT. The rate of breast cancer recurrence was 17 per 1,000 person years in the users, versus 30 per 1,000 in the non-users, RR = 0.5. Breast cancer mortality was five per 1,000 women years in hormone users, and 15 per 1,000 in non-users, RR = 0.34 {111}. They concluded that HRT after breast cancer does not seem to increase recurrences or increase mortality. In a short study of 125 hormone users matched to 363 non-users there were 15 deaths in hormone users versus 134 in non-users; 12% versus 37%. In another study one new cancer occurred in 39 estrogen users and 14 developed cancer in the 280 non-users; 2.55% versus 5% {167}.

The above studies indicate that ET/EPT can be offered to women as evidence has accumulated regarding the safety of hormone use {44,88}. Women who develop breast cancer can be offered estrogen treatment for menopausal symptoms and protection against osteoporosis after a thorough discussion of all available data; informed consent should be obtained.

Conclusion

Breast cancer is being diagnosed in early stages, and the survival rates have increased due to early diagnosis and treatment. Women lead normal lives for many years. They need to be given the opportunity to benefit from all available treatment. Estrogen replacement can be used for severe symptoms in breast cancer survivors after thorough explanation, and understanding, of benefits and risks.

TABLE 23.1: INCIDENCE OF BREAST CANCER AT WILFORD HALL USAF MEDICAL CENTER 1975–1983

Therapy Group	Patient-Years of Ovservation	Patients with Cancer	Incidence (Per 100,000)
Estrogen—Progestogen Users	16,466	11	66.8
Unopposed Estrogen Users	19,676	28	142.3
Estrogen Vaginal Cream Users	4,298	5	116.3
Progestogen Users	1,825	3	164.4
Non-Users	6,404	22	343.5
TOTAL	48,669	68	141.8

FIGURE 23.1—Incidence of Cancer by Age

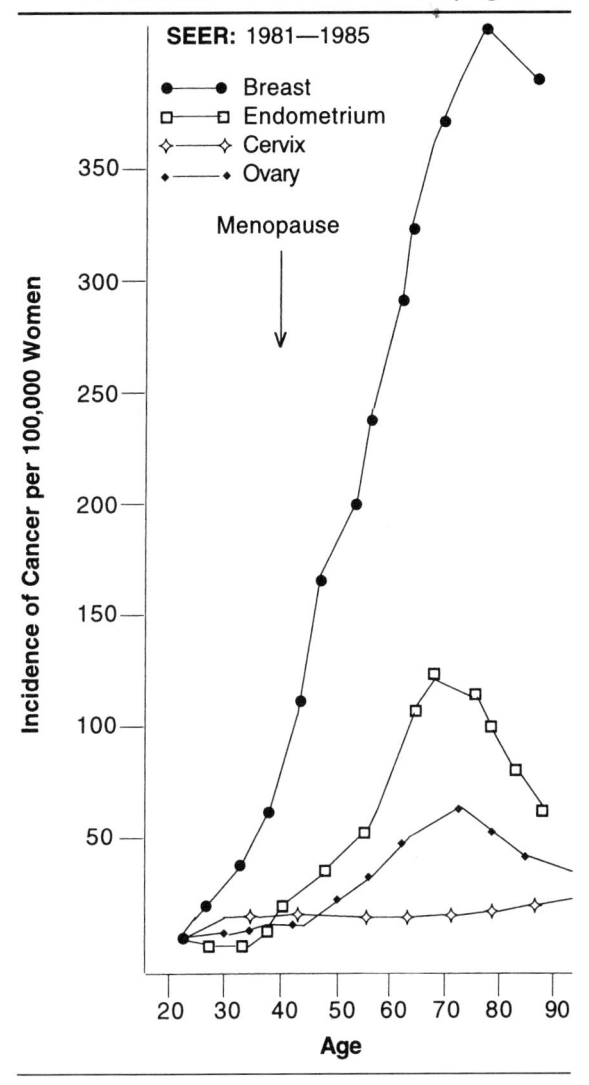

Incidence of breast, endometrial, cervical and ovarian cancer in women by age.

FIGURE 23.2—Incidence of Breast Cancer

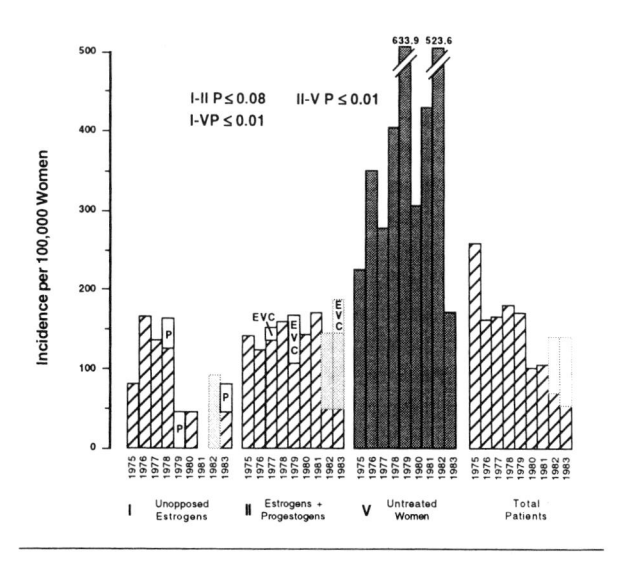

Incidence of breast cancer in the various treatment groups compared with untreated from 1975–1983. {46}

FIGURE 23.3—Incidence of Breast Cancer Compared to Number of Estrogen and Estrogen-Progesten Treated Women

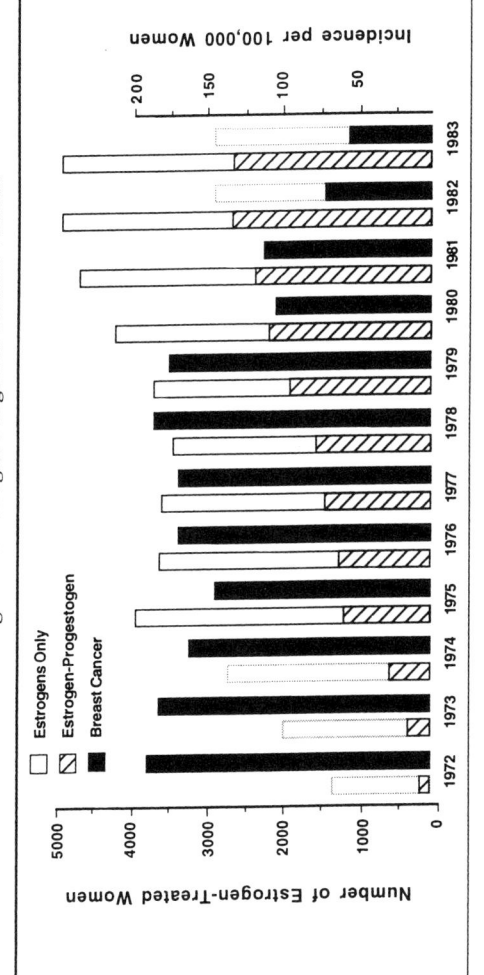

Comparison of the number of estrogen and estrogen-progestogen users with the incidence of breast cancer by year over the period 1972–1983. Solid lines indicate prospective and follow-up study and broken lines illustrate retrospective data, while semi-broken lines (1982–1983) indicate cancer in past users. {46}

SECTION 24: THROMBOEMBOLIC DISEASE

Clinical Information

Estrogen replacement therapy has been thought to increase thromboembolic phenomena, which are listed as contraindications. This concept is largely based on observations suggesting an association between oral contraceptives and vascular thrombosis. Despite a positive association between aging and thromboembolic complications, clinical studies have failed to observe any increased risk of these disorders {103,110}. In the recent studies from WHI and HERS the incidence of thromboembolism seemed to increase by two-fold {77,131}.

Coagulation changes that occur with aging include:
- Increase in factor V
- Increase in factor VII
- Possible increase in factor VIII
- No change in antithrombin III

Coagulation changes that occur with estrogen replacement include:
- Increase in fibrinogen (still within normal range)
- Slight decrease in antithrombin III (still within normal range)
- Decrease in factor V
- No change in factors VII or X
- No change in prothrombin time or partial thromboplastin time

Research

Deaths from cerebral vascular accidents (CVA) declined from an expected 15 to eight during estrogen therapy over a 15-year period of treatment {11}. It was concluded that estrogens delay aging of the arteries.

In the most recent study, protection from stroke was observed in all age groups except the youngest RR = 0.53;

95% CI, 0.31 to 0.91 {114}. This was unaffected by possible confounding variables such as:
- Smoking
- Alcohol intake
- Body mass
- Exercise

Another study found a significantly lower incidence of stroke syndromes in long-term estrogen users compared with a similar group who had not used estrogens {64}. No significant difference in the incidence of either thrombophlebitis or embolism was observed between estrogen-treated women and patients who had never received estrogens. In a double-blind study, thrombophlebitis occurred in 13 of 84 estrogen-progestogen users and 17 of 84 placebo users {103}. Only one incidence of pulmonary embolism was encountered during the 10 years of this study, and it occurred in a placebo user.

Estrogen labeling has been recently changed so that no longer are all thromboembolic events contraindications. Active thrombophlebitis or thromboembolic disorders remain contraindications as do histories of thrombophlebitis, thrombosis, or thromboembolic disorders associated with previous estrogen use. No longer are postpartum, postoperative, or traumatic blood clots contraindications. However, in patients with any history of thromboembolic disease, it would seem prudent to obtain coagulation studies before therapy and repeat these after three to six months of estrogen use.

SECTION 25: HYPERTENSION

Research

Because the original high-dose oral contraceptives caused transient hypertension in some young women, estrogen replacement therapy has been expected to have a similar effect. However, numerous studies have indicated that estrogen therapy has a beneficial effect on hypertension.

Some of these studies and their findings include:
- Duke University—Incidence of new hypertensive cardiovascular disease of 16.3 percent in estrogen-treated women vs 31.7 percent in nonusers ($P \leq 0.001$) {65}
- Southern California—Study of 1,496 women, after adjusting for effects of obesity, found estrogen-treated women tended to have lower blood pressure and blood glucose than controls {6}
- Wilford Hall—Estrogen users had lower diastolic blood pressures (BPs) than other groups; nonusers were more obese ($P \leq 0.05$) {46}
- Australian studies observed lowered systolic BPs with one natural estrogen—*Ogen*—and lowered diastolic BPs with another—*Premarin* {175}
- An English study observed that both systolic and diastolic BPs are significantly reduced in women on various regimens of hormone replacement {90}.

Hypertension increases in the age group of postmenopausal women. Therefore, cases will be found among these estrogen users {114,156}. However, these do not establish the role of estrogens in hypertension. Elevations in BPs can coexist with hormone replacement, therefore, blood pressure should be routinely monitored.

Other studies have reported on the effect of estrogen use on the renin-aldosterone system. One study showed no activation of the renin-aldosterone system in patients using estradiol valerate therapy {123}. Another study reported an increased plasma renin activity in users of conjugated estrogens, but no effect on the renin concentration itself. There are no adverse effects of estrogens on blood pressures when hormone users were matched to controls and corrected for age and weight.

Recommendations for Treatment

If hypertension does occur in estrogen users, estrogen replacement does not have to stop {123}. Instead, as a step, salt intake should be restricted to 3,000 mg daily. If salt restriction alone does not control the hypertension, a mild anti-hypertensive, such as hydrochlorothiazide, at 25 to 50 mg daily, can be added. Only if these two measures fail to improve blood pressure levels should there be consideration of ending estrogen replacement. Most hypertensive patients require less medication after hormone replacement.

25.

SECTION 26: GALLBLADDER DISEASE

Research

Some studies have indicated that estrogen replacement therapy increases the risk of gallbladder disease, especially cholelithiasis. The liver responds to oral estrogens by an increase in sex hormone binding globulin (SHBG). It has been suggested that oral estrogens may affect the liver's excretory functions and increase the incidence of gallstones.

Gallstones seem to occur more frequently in the silent form. In one study, oral cholecystography showed that 5.1 percent of those tested had gallstones present {132}. Silent cases occurred twice as often, and the diet was not significantly different in those with or without gallstones.

Studies reported that the risk of surgically confirmed gallbladder disease increased 2.5 times with estrogen therapy {11}. While in others the risk of cholesterol cholelithiasis was increased by both estrogens and obesity {74}. Both factors operated independently, with estrogen increasing the risk of gallstones at all weight levels. However, in the Duke University study, new occurrence of gallbladder disease was significantly lower ($P \leq 0.05$) in the estrogen users compared with controls {64}. At the end of a 10-year New York study, the estrogen-progestogen group had a higher, although statistically insignificant, incidence of cholelithiasis {103}.

The most recent study found no increased risk for gallstones among estrogen users RR=1.18; 95% CI, 0.65 to 2.13 {81}. Among estrogen users, the duration of use was similar in cases and controls.

Recommendations for Treatment

Since it is not feasible to screen all postmenopausal women for occult gallbladder disease prior to estrogen therapy, it has been suggested that patients should be instructed regarding the early signs of cholelithiasis {74}, including:
- Right upper quadrant pain
- Indigestion
- Eructation
- Nausea

NOTES

SECTION 27: NUTRITION AND DIET

A healthy lifestyle is very important for postmenopausal women. Remaining active, not smoking, choosing the right foods, and not gaining weight help prevent cardiovascular diseases and decrease other problems of aging. Estrogen replacement therapy, as important as it is, should not be a substitute for a healthy lifestyle.

Body Weight

It is commonly thought that menopause, estrogen therapy, and even hysterectomy cause women to gain weight. This is just not true. What happens to cause some women to gain weight is that, at menopause, metabolism decreases. Some cannot continue to eat the same this year as last year because of decreased metabolism.

In the three-year PEPI trial all 875 healthy, postmenopausal women gained weight. The greatest weight gain was in the placebo group, which had an average weight gain of 4.6 pounds, compared to the estrogen user group, which had an average weight gain of 1.5 pounds.

A healthy lifestyle becomes even more important after menopause. Smoking decreases the good HDL cholesterol, which aids in removal of cholesterol from the blood. Increased activity, such as long, brisk walks, increases HDL cholesterol. Strategies for keeping cholesterol low and remaining healthy are to:

- Reduce the amount of total and saturated fat and cholesterol in the diet
- Use monounsaturated oils instead of saturated fats
- Eat foods high in soluble fiber, e.g., oat bran
- Eat foods high in beta carotene and other antioxidants
- Drink coffee in moderation
- Limit the amount of salt in the diet
- Eat calcium-rich foods (see Section 20)

Fat Grams

Counting calories from fat is not only most important for losing and maintaining weight, but also is the best diet method for lowering cholesterol and triglyceride levels. This recent advance has been a major breakthrough in weight reduction. Calories from fat grams are far more important than total calories in the diet. For women, restricting the diet to no more than 20 to 25 fat grams per day can result in a one- to three-pound weight loss each week. The T-Factor Diet {84} is an excellent source for determining fat grams in foods and recipes and general instructions on how to lose and maintain weight.

The low carbohydrate *Atkins Diet* is effective and weight loss is more rapid than counting fat grams. It takes more calories to metabolize protein than it does carbohydrates. However, it may increase acidosis and triglycerides, which can be dangerous. High triglycerides not only increase heart disease in women, but can also lead to acute hemorrhagic pancreatitis.

27.

SECTION 28: LIPID METABOLISM

Changes in Blood Lipid Profile

Both surgical and natural menopause appear to be related to adverse changes in blood lipid profile. These changes include:
- Development of atherosclerosis at an earlier age
- Increased hypertension
- Increased incidence of coronary artery disease

Natural Estrogens

Low dosages of natural estrogens increase HDL cholesterol with corresponding decreases in both LDL and very low density lipoproteins (VLDL), an antiatherogenic pattern.

Transdermal estradiol and subcutaneous estradiol pellets also increase HDL cholesterol, but seem to take longer than oral estrogens because they avoid the first liver-pass. In a comparative study between estradiol pellets and transdermal estradiol, there was a significant increase in HDL cholesterol with the pellets after 12 weeks; it took 24 weeks for the patch to increase HDL significantly {148}. The total cholesterol-to-HDL ratio was also significantly decreased at 12 weeks with pellets but took 24 weeks with the patch.

In the Coronary Drug Project, high dosages of conjugated estrogens (5 to 15 mg) had the opposite effect of lower dosages, resulting in an atherogenic pattern of decreased HDL with corresponding increases of both LDL and VLDL {158}.

Birth Control Pills

Moderate-to-high dosage oral contraceptives, e.g., 50 µg of ethinyl estradiol, increase both HDL and VLDL. However, when the 19-nor-testosterone progestogens are added, the atherogenic pattern develops with a decrease in HDL, while LDL and VLDL both increase. HDL is further decreased by smoking and results in a relative risk of 2.5 for heart disease mortality {97}. The newer low-dosage oral contraceptives do not have an adverse effect on lipid metabolism.

FIGURE 28.1— Changes in Lipoproteins

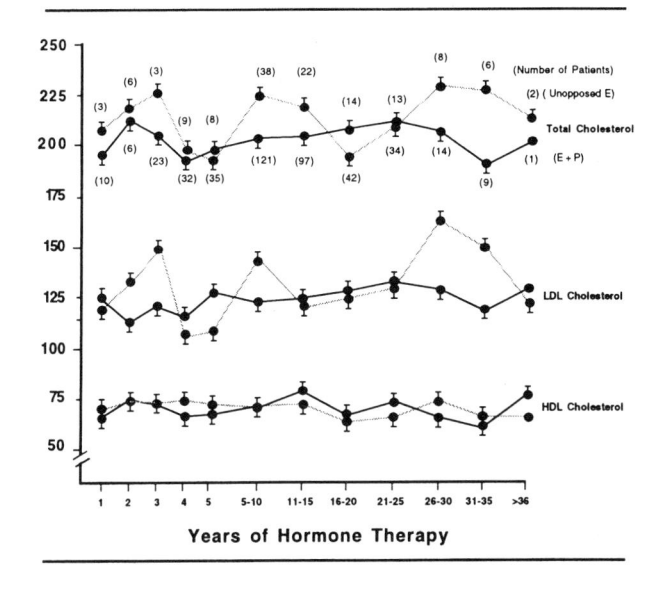

Mean values of total cholesterol, LDL cholesterol, and HDL cholesterol compared in the unopposed estrogen users (unopposed E) to the estrogen-progestogen users (E + P) from one to 44 years of hormone replacement therapy. (Reproduced from Gambrell and Teran with permission of the publisher) {53}.

Added Progestogens

Although natural estrogens increase HDL cholesterol, concern has been expressed that added progestogens may negate this beneficial effect. Most of this concern is based on short-term studies of estrogen-progestogen use that have not been confirmed in studies of more than 12 months' duration {6,53}.

In one such study {6,53}:
- HDL was significantly increased and LDL significantly decreased in both unopposed estrogen users and estrogen-progestogen users

- Triglycerides were significantly increased in unopposed estrogen users but not different from controls in estrogen-progestogen users

This shows that added progestogens may actually benefit the lipid pattern by minimizing the increase in triglycerides usually seen with estrogen therapy. This was confirmed in a large study of 4,958 postmenopausal women where it was also observed that estrogen users had higher levels of apolipoprotein A-1 than non-users {102}.

Another study evaluated different dosages of *Estrace* using a standard dosage of progestogen, 1 mg of norethindrone acetate for 11 days. The study found:
- A dose-related increase in HDL
- 4 mg ↑ HDL <2 mg <1 mg *Estrace*
- Significant decrease in LDL with all three dosages
- Norethindrone acetate did not negate the increase in HDL or decrease in LDL

The three-year PEPI trail concluded that estrogen alone, or in combination with the progestogen, improves lipoprotein levels and lowers fibrinogen levels without detectable effects on post-challenge insulin or blood pressure. Unopposed estrogen produced the greatest increase in HDL cholesterol, but there was a high incidence of endometrial hyperplasia. Conjugated estrogens with cyclic medroxyprogesterone acetate had the most favorable effect on HDL cholesterol without any risk of endometrial hyperplasia.

Over the long-term there are no adverse effects on lipids of added progestogens to estrogen replacement. In a long-term study, the only significant changes were related to obesity (↑ triglycerides) and smoking (↓ HDL) {53}. In this cross-sectional study at the Medical College of Georgia:
- 556 were postmenopausal women
- 132 were using unopposed estrogen
- 424 were using estrogen and progestogen
- The age range was 44 to 85 years, with a mean age of 57.14 ± 10.56 years
- Duration of therapy was from one to 44 years, with a mean duration of 11.97 ± 8.11 years

Figure 28.1 shows the mean values from one to more than 36 years of hormone replacement. Total cholesterol hovered around 200 to 210 mg/dL in both unopposed estrogen users and estrogen-progestogen users. LDL ranged from 110 to 130 mg/dL in both groups (normal range 86 to 138). There were no differences in mean HDL, ranging from 60 to 70 mg/dL (average risk 54 to 59; low risk 59 to 74). There were no significant differences in mean HDL among unopposed estrogen users (67.0 ± 3.94), estrogen plus C-21 progestogen users (64.5 ± 4.16), and estrogen plus C-19 progestogen users (61.9 ± 3.84).

Even androgens do not adversely affect lipids when adequate dosages of estrogen are given, since 84.2 percent of these patients also received androgens, usually in the form of testosterone pellets.

The tremendous benefit of preventing cardiovascular disease with hormone replacement therapy cannot be fully explained by the changes in lipid patterns {133}. Other factors have roles such as direct effects of estrogens on arterial walls, since estrogen receptors have been identified in coronary vessels.

Estrogens may:

- Improve vascular blood flow, even dilatation of coronary arteries
- Decrease platelet adhesiveness
- Increase endothelial-derived relaxing factor (EDRF)
- Be mediated through prostacyclin and thromboxane metabolism
- Increase cardiac output
- Reduce vascular resistance
- Increase velocity of blood flow
- Inhibit atherosclerosis progression
- Inhibit coronary thrombosis

SECTION 29: MANAGEMENT OF SIDE EFFECTS

Resumption of Menses

In postmenopausal women treated with combination estrogen-progestogen therapy, withdrawal bleeding occurs in as many as 97 percent until age 60, decreasing to 60 percent after age 65.

Generally, patient acceptance of resumption of menses has been good if the relative benefits and risks are carefully explained. These include:
- The reduced incidence of endometrial cancer (see Section 22)
- No increased risk of breast cancer; in some women, added progestogen reduces its incidence (see Section 23)
- Promotion of new bone formation, helping restore bone that has been lost to osteoporosis (see Section 5)

In addition, the menses often change for the better. Frequently, the menses:
- Are lighter
- Are less painful
- Have less abnormal bleeding

Patients most reluctant to resume menses are those who experienced adverse menstrual effects. After menopause, withdrawal menses from hormone therapy are usually:
- Only three to four days in duration
- Free of dysmenorrhea
- Without premenstrual syndrome (PMS) symptoms

In one study {51}, abnormal bleeding requiring curettage occurred in:
- 23.3 percent of nonusers of hormones
- 14 percent of unopposed estrogen users
- Only 3.9 percent of estrogen-progestogen users

In addition, the estrogen-progestogen users need not have the annual endometrial biopsies that are recommended for all unopposed estrogen users with intact uteri (see Section 11).

For those patients who cannot tolerate resumption of menses, cyclic combined estrogen-progestogen therapy is an alternative that will produce amenorrhea in 75 percent of patients after four to six months (see Section 17).

Side Effects of Estrogens

Side effects of estrogens may include:
- Breast tenderness
- Edema or bloating
- PMS-like symptoms
- Nausea
- Headaches

Most patients have few, if any, side effects from estrogen replacement. If side effects occur, they are minimal and transient {47}.

Breast tenderness and sometimes slight breast enlargement may occur during the first two to three months after initiation of therapy. Mastodynia usually abates with time, and reassurance is often all that patients need.

If breast tenderness persists, the estrogen dosage can be reduced if more than 0.625 mg conjugated estrogens were prescribed. However, this should be the lowest dosage in order to prevent osteoporosis (see Section 5).

Adding a progestogen to estrogen therapy reduces breast tenderness in time, although it may initially aggravate breast tenderness. Reassurance to patients is often all that is needed. Adding androgens to estrogen therapy or to estrogen-progestogen therapy may also ameliorate breast tenderness.

A mild diuretic, such as hydrochlorothiazide or spironolactone (25 to 50 mg), will relieve symptoms caused by estrogen-related fluid retention, such as:
- Edema
- Bloating
- Abdominal pressure

- Breast tenderness
- PMS-like symptoms (headache, irritability)

The diuretic is usually given seven to ten days before menses during the days of added progestogen. A change to a different estrogen is sometimes necessary (see Table 14.1) or a change in the route of administration, e.g., the transdermal estrogen, may help.

Nausea is rare in the low dosages of estrogen usually required for estrogen replacement. If nausea persists after two months of therapy, a change of estrogens or the route of administration may help.

Headaches are generally relieved by estrogen replacement. Most headaches are transient and respond to analgesics. Others may occur only with cyclic therapy on the days at the end of the month when estrogens are not taken. Estrogens can be taken continuously as long as they are opposed with progestogens for 13 days each month. Usually, migraine headaches diminish at menopause and sometimes recur with estrogen replacement. Sometimes headaches respond to a mild diuretic, but it may be necessary to add an androgen to the estrogen therapy. The best response is offered by combination products such as:
- *Estratest* (orally)
- *Depo-Testadiol* (by injection)
- Estradiol-testosterone pellets

Side Effects of Progestogens

Side effects of progestogens include:
- PMS-like symptoms
- Lethargy
- Depression and irritability
- Abdominal bloating
- Breast tenderness

Mild PMS-like symptoms usually respond to a diuretic such as hydrochlorothiazide or spironolactone at 25 to 50 mg for seven to ten days before menses. If this is ineffective, a change should be made to another oral progestogen.

Breast tenderness may be initiated, aggravated, or relieved when progestogens are added to estrogen replacement. Symptoms usually abate after three to six months. If mastodynia persists, a change should be made to another progestogen (see Table 17.1). For some women, C-21 progestogens such as medroxyprogesterone acetate are better than 19-nor-testosterone progestogens such as norethindrone acetate; for others, the reverse is true.

In a rare case, a woman may experience side effects with all oral progestogens. Progesterone vaginal suppositories (25 to 50 mg) or oral micronized progesterone (100 to 300 mg) often eliminate these reactions.

SECTION 30: CONTRAINDICATIONS

Contraindications for Estrogens

The following contraindications are listed in the product literature for most estrogens:
- Known or suspected cancer of the breast
- Known or suspected estrogen-dependent neoplasia
- Known or suspected pregnancy
- Undiagnosed abnormal genital bleeding
- Active thrombophlebitis or thromboembolic disorders

Women on estrogen replacement therapy have not been reported to have an increased risk of thrombophlebitis and/or thromboembolic disease. However, there is insufficient information regarding women who have had previous thromboembolic disease.

There is no evidence that estrogen replacement increases the risk for breast cancer. However, estrogen is the growth hormone of mammary tissue, and many physicians consider it a contraindication.

Four prominent gynecologic oncologists now recommend that patients with successfully treated breast cancer be allowed to use hormone replacement, since there are no data indicating it worsens prognosis {30,34,35,40,150}. Theoretically, estrogen receptors in carcinoma of the breast would allow selection of some patients for estrogen replacement, yet only 50 percent of estrogen receptor positive tumors will respond either to endocrine ablative surgery or anti-estrogen therapy. When progesterone receptors in mammary cancer are also positive, this predictive response increases to 70 percent. There are now more than sixty studies that show it is safe to give estrogen replacement to patients with previous breast cancer (see Sections 8 and 23) {88}.

Endometrial cancer may not have to remain a strict contraindication. Gynecologic oncologists at Wilford Hall USAF Medical Center provided estrogen replacement in women with Stage I well differentiated adenocarcinoma of the endometrium, since there was little likelihood of metastases.

The five-year survival rate was in excess of 96.7 percent. A study from Duke University indicated that prognosis was actually improved in endometrial cancer patients treated with estrogens {31}.

Any abnormal postmenopausal bleeding should be thoroughly evaluated (see Section 11). Once malignancy is excluded and endometrial hyperplasia has been adequately treated with progestogens (see Section 21), estrogen-progestogen therapy can be safely administered.

Although there is no evidence that low dosages of natural estrogens have any adverse effects on coagulation factors or thromboembolic disease (see Section 24) estrogen replacement should be given cautiously to women who had blood clots previously while using estrogens. Thromboembolic events not related to a history of hormone use no longer are contraindications for replacement therapy.

Contraindications for Progestogens

The following contraindications are listed in the product literature for most progestogens:
- A past or present history of:
  - Thrombophlebitis
  - Thromboembolic disorders
  - Cerebral apoplexy
- Liver dysfunction or disease
- Known or suspected carcinoma of the breast
- Undiagnosed vaginal bleeding
- Missed abortion
- As a diagnostic test for pregnancy

Almost identical contraindications are listed for progestogens as for estrogens, even though there is no evidence that progestogens have any adverse effect on coagulation factors or thromboembolic disorders. However, this labeling should not preclude physicians from using their best judgments in the interest of their patients.

If liver function studies are normal, patients with histories of liver dysfunction or disease can safely be given progestogens. However, liver function studies should be repeated after three to six months of progestogen therapy.

There is no evidence that progestogens increase the risk for breast cancer. There is, in fact, increasing evidence that adding progestogens to estrogen replacement may decrease the risk for carcinoma of the breast in some women, and that long-term progesterone deficiency can increase the risk for breast cancer (see Section 23) {28,29}. For medical and/or legal reasons, prescribing progestogens to breast cancer patients other than for treatment of metastatic carcinoma of the breast with megestrol acetate is hazardous in the United States.

In addition to megestrol acetate, medroxyprogesterone acetate is also used to treat metastatic breast carcinoma in Canada and Europe and is just beginning to be used in the United States {13,75}. Comparative trials between tamoxifen and medroxyprogesterone acetate indicate that progestogens are just as effective in the treatment of metastatic breast cancer as the weak estrogen tamoxifen {13}.

One of the most effective therapies for Stage IV metastatic carcinoma of the breast at the MD Anderson Cancer Center was a combination of estrogen and progestogen {75}. Seven days of estrogen were given to enhance progesterone receptors in mammary cancer cells, followed by 21 days of high-dose medroxyprogesterone acetate for 21 days in repeated cycles. The objective remission response was 56.7 percent for up to six years, with a mean duration of 22 months. Yet it is ironic that this progestogen, as well as all other progestogens except megestrol acetate, remain listed as contraindicated for women with breast cancer in the United States.

Undiagnosed genital bleeding becomes apparent in the course of proper evaluation of postmenopausal women (see Section 11). Endometrial hyperplasia should be treated with progestogens to prevent adenocarcinoma of the endometrium.

NOTES

SECTION 31: ALTERNATIVE THERAPY

Clinical Information

Estrogens and progestogens are always the preferred hormone replacement treatment since they:
- Relieve menopausal symptoms
- Prevent the metabolic consequences (osteoporosis and atherosclerosis) of long-term estrogen deficiency

If estrogens are contraindicated, progestogens cannot be used since the contraindications are identical (see Section 30). Alternative therapies are available to treat menopausal symptoms, including:
- Vasomotor symptoms
- Urogenital atrophy
- Psychogenic manifestations
- Osteoporosis

Vasomotor Symptoms

Androgens are effective in relieving such symptoms as:
- Hot flushes (or flashes)
- Night sweats
- Psychogenic manifestations

Any of the oral androgens such as methyltestosterone 5 mg (see Table 16.1) or injectables such as Depo-Testosterone (50 mg every four weeks) can be used. However, androgens do not prevent atrophic vaginitis or coronary artery disease, and they are probably ineffective in preventing osteoporosis in the dosages that can be given to postmenopausal women.

Bellergal-S is a tablet combining phenobarbital, ergotamine, and belladonna alkaloids given in a dosage of one tablet twice daily. It is effective for:
- Reducing hot flushes (or flashes)
- Reducing night sweats
- Helping to calm restlessness
- Relieving insomnia

Clonidine HCl is an antihypertensive agent effective for hot flushes. The dosage is 0.1 mg three times daily.

Urogenital Atrophy

No good alternative to estrogen is available for treatment of atrophic vaginitis. If oral estrogens are contraindicated, so are estrogen vaginal creams, which are well absorbed through the vaginal mucosa. Local antibiotics will treat infections, and one- to two-percent testosterone cream is effective for kraurosis vulvae.

Surgical lubricants can be prescribed for dyspareunia.

Psychogenic Manifestations

Alternative therapies available for treatment of psychogenic manifestations include:
- Tranquilizers
- Androgens
- Calcium channel blockers

Tranquilizers can be used to treat depression and restlessness, but they are not good substitutes for estrogen replacement since they do not prevent effects of menopausal estrogen deprivation.

Androgens are most effective when they can be prescribed along with estrogens. Used alone, androgens still offer:
- Treatment of disturbances of the libido
- Promotion of a sense of well-being
- Partial relief of depression

A calcium channel blocker (*Calan*–Pharmacia) can be fairly effective in relieving headaches. It works best when combined with estrogen replacement but, can be effective used alone. The dosage is titrated, starting with 80 mg daily and increasing every week to a maximum of four times daily until headaches are blocked. Triptains, namely *Imitrex, Maxalt, Relpax* and *Zomig,* have been used successfully in migraine headaches.

Osteoporosis and Atherosclerosis

When estrogens are contraindicated, calcium supplementation should be increased to 1,500 to 2,000 mg daily (see Section 20). There is some evidence that calcium alone will help prevent osteoporosis and reduce fracture rate {125}, although this has recently been questioned. It is best to provide estrogen replacement whenever possible.

There have been several agents approved for prevention of osteoporosis. *Alendronate* has been used the longest and is available in daily or once-a-week dosage. *Residronate* is another bisphosphonate with good results. *Calcitonin* nasal spray and human parathormone, and raloxifene are also available for prevention and treatment of osteoporosis.

There is really no alternative to estrogen replacement for prevention of atherosclerosis. Good nutrition is advisable to reduce dietary intake of cholesterol (see Section 27). Other measures include increases in physical activities, e.g., jogging or brisk walking.

NOTES

SECTION 32: REFERENCES

1. Adams MR, Washburn SA, Wagner JD, et al: Arterial changes: Estrogen deficiency and effects of hormone replacement. In: Treatment of the Postmenopausal Woman: Basic and Clinical Aspects, RA Lobo (ed). New York, Raven Press, 1994, pp 243–250.

2. American-Canadian Cooperative Study Group: Persantine aspirin trial in cerebral ischemia-Part III: Risk factor for stroke. Stroke 1986; 17:12.

3. Anderson E, Hamburger S, Lin JH, et al: Characteristics of menopausal women seeking assistance. Am J Obstet Gynecol 1987; 156:428.

4. Annual Cancer Statistics Review: NIH Publication No. 88–2789. Bethesda, National Institutes of Health, 1987, p 111.36.

5. Barrett-Conner E, Brown V, Turner J, et al: Heart disease risk factors and hormone use in postmenopausal women. JAMA 1978; 241:2167.

6. Barrett-Conner E, Wingard DL, Criqui MH: Postmenopausal estrogen use and heart disease risk factors in the 1980s. JAMA 1989; 261:2095.

7. Bergkvist L, Adami H-O, Persson I, et al: Prognosis after breast cancer diagnosis in women exposed to estrogen and estrogen-progestogen replacement therapy. Am J Epidemiol 1989; 130:221–228.

8. Birge SJ: The role of estrogen deficiency in the aging central nervous system. In: Treatment of the Postmenopausal Woman: Basic and Clinical Aspects, RA Lobo, (ed). New York, Raven Press, 1994, pp 153–157.

9. Block DM, Thompson DE, Bauer DC. Fracture risk reduction with alendronate in women with osteoporosis: The fracture intervention trial. FIT research group. J Clin Endocrinol Metab 2000: 85(11) 4118–4124.

10. Brenner DE, Kukull WA, Stergachis A, et al: Postmenopausal estrogen replacement therapy and the risk of Alzheimer's disease: A population-based case-control study. Am J Epidemiol 1994; 140–262.

11. Burch JC, Byrd BF, Vaughn WK: Results of estrogen treatment in one thousand hysterectomized women for 14,318 years. In: Consensus on Menopausal Research. Van Keep PA, Greenblatt RB, Albeaux-Fernet M (eds.) Lancaster, England: MTP Press Ltd., 1976;164–169.

12. Bush TL, Whiteman M, Flaws JA: Hormone replacement therapy and breast cancer: a qualitative analysis. Obstet Gynecol 2001; 98:498–508

13. Buzdar AU. Progestins in cancer treatment. In: Endocrine Management of Cancer. Stoll, BA (ed.) Basel, Switzerland: Karger, 1988;1–15.

14. Cameron ST, Critchley HOD, Glassier AF, et al: Continuous transdermal oestrogen and interrupted progestogen as a novel bleed-free regimen of hormone replacement therapy for postmenopausal women. Br J Obstet Gynaecol 1997; 104: 1184–1190.

15. Campbell S, Whitehead M: Oestrogen therapy and the menopausal syndrome. In: Clinics in Obstetrics and Gynecology. Greenblatt RB, Studd JWW (eds.) London, England: WB Saunders Co., Ltd., 1977:31.

16. Casper RF: Estrogen with interrupted progestin HRT: a review of experimental and clinical evidence. Maturitas 2000; 34:97–108.

17. Chen W, Colditz G, Rosner B et al: Use of postmenopausal hormones, alcohol, and risk for invasive breast cancer. Annals of Internal Medicine Nov 2002; 137:798–804.

18. Chestnut CH III, Silverman S, Andriano K et al: A randomized trial of nasal spray salmon calcitonin in post menopausal women with established osteoporosis: the prevent recurrence of osteoporotic fractures study. Proof study group. Am J Med 2000: 109 (4) 267–276.

19. Chetkowski RJ, Meldrum DR, Steingold KA, et al: Biologic effects of transdermal estradiol. N Engl J Med 1986; 314:1615.

20. Cobleigh MA, Berris RF, Bush T, et al: Estrogen replacement therapy in breast cancer survivors: A time for change. JAMA 1994; 272:540–545.

21. Col NF, Hirota LK, Orr RK et al: Hormone replacement therapy after breast cancer. A systematic review and quantitative assessment of risk. J Clin Oncol 2001;19:2357–2363.

22. Col NF, Pomker SG, Goldberg RG: Individualizing therapy to prevent long-term consequences of estrogen deficiency in post menopausal women. Arch Interm Med 1999; 159:1458–66.

23. Colditz GA, Hankinson SE, Hunter DJ et al: The use of estrogens and progestins and the risk of breast cancer in postmenopausal women. N Engl J Med 1995; 332: 1589–1593.

24. Colditz GA, Egan KM, Stampfer MJ: Hormone replacement therapy and risk of breast cancer: Results from epidemiologic studies. Am J Obstet Gynecol 1993; 168:1473–1480.

25. Collaborative Group on Hormonal Factors in Breast Cancer: Breast cancer and hormone replacement therapy: Collaborative reanalysis of data from 51 epidemiological studies of 52,705 women with breast cancer and 108,411 women without breast cancer. Lancet 1997; 350:1047–1059.

26. Collaborative Group on Hormonal Factors in Breast Cancer: Breast cancer and hormonal contraceptives: further results. Contraception 1996; 54: 1–106.

27. Comerci JT Jr, Fields AL, Runowitz LD, Goldbert GL. Continuous low-dose combined hormonal replacement therapy and the risk of endometrial cancer. Gynecol Oncol 1997; 64:425.

28. Coulam CB, Annegers JF: Chronic anovulation risk may increase postmenopausal breast cancer risk. JAMA 1983;249:445–446.

29. Cowan LD, Gordis L, Tonascia JA, et al: Breast cancer incidence in women with a history of progesterone deficiency. Am J Epidemiol 1981; 114:209–217.

30. Creasman WT: Estrogen replacement therapy. Is previously treated cancer a contraindication? Obstet Gynecol 1991; 77:308–312.

31. Creasman WT, Henderson D, Hindshaw W, et al. Estrogen replacement therapy in the patient treated for endometrial cancer. Obstet Gynecol 1986; 67:326.

32. Darj E, Nilsson S, Axelsson O, et al: Clinical and endometrial effects of estradiol and progesterone in postmenopausal women. Maturitas 1991; 13:109.

33. Dennerstein L, Laby B, Burrows GD, et al: Headache and sex hormone therapy. Headache 1978;18:146.

34. Dew J, Eden J, Beller E, Magarey C, Schwartz P., et al: A cohort study of hormone replacement therapy given to women previously treated for breast cancer. Climacteric 1998; 1:137–142.

35. DiSaia P, Brewster W, Ziotas A, Anton-Culver H: Breast cancer survival and hormone replacement therapy: a cohort analysis. Am J Clin Oncol 2000;23: 541–545.

36. DiSaia PJ, Creasman WT, Odicino F, et al: Hormone replacement therapy in breast cancer. Lancet 1993; 324:1232.

37. DiSaia PJ, Grosen EA, Kurosaki T, Gildea M, Cowan B, Anton-Culver H: Hormone replacement therapy in breast cancer survivors; a cohort study. Am J Obstet Gynecol 1996; 174:1494–1498.

38. Doren M, Schneider HPG: Long-term compliance of continuous combined estrogen and progestogen replacement in postmenopausal women. Maturitas 1996;25:99.

39. Ebeling PR, Altey LM, Guthrie JR et al: Bone turnover markers and bone density across the menopausal transition. J Clin Endocr Metab 1996;81:3366.

40. Eden JA, Bush T, Nard S, et al: A case-controlled study of combined continuous estrogen-progestin replacement therapy among women with a personal history of breast cancer: Menopause. J N Am Menopause Soc 1995;2:67–72.

41. Ettinger B, Black DM, Mikak BH et al: Reduction of vertebral fracture risk in post menopausal women with osteoporosis treated with raloxifene: results from 3 year randomized clinical trial. Multiple Outcomes Raloxifene Evaluation. (MORE) Investigations. JAMA 1999: 287:637–645.

42. Ewertz M: Influence of noncontraceptive exogenous and endogenous sex hormones in breast cancer risks in Denmark. Int J Cancer 1988;42:832–838.

43. Gambrell RD Jr: Proposal to decrease the risk and improve the prognosis of breast cancer. Am J Obstet Gynecol 1984;150:119–132.

44. Gambrell RD Jr: Sex steroids and cancer. Obstet Gynecol Clin N Am 1987;14:191–206.

45. Gambrell RD Jr: The menopause: Benefits and risks of estrogen-progestogen replacement therapy. Fertil Steril 1982;37:457–474.

46. Gambrell RD Jr: Use of progestogen therapy. Am J Obstet Gynecol 1987;156:1304–1313.

47. Gambrell RD Jr: Management of hormone replacement side effects: Menopause. J N Am Menopause Soc 1994;1:67–72.

48. Gambrell RD Jr: Hormone replacement therapy and breast cancer risk. Arch Fam Med 1996;5:341–348.

49. Gambrell RD Jr: Strategies to reduce the incidence of endometrial cancer in postmenopausal women. Am J Obstet Gynecol 1997;177:1196–1203.

50. Gambrell RD Jr, Cherry JK, Davis DL, et al: (Letter) Mammography screening. JAMA 1994;271:1827.

51. Gambrell RD Jr, Castaneda TA, Ricci CA: Management of postmenopausal bleeding to prevent endometrial cancer. Maturitas 1978;1:99–106.

52. Gambrell RD Jr, McDonough PG: The "red queen" and endometrial hyperplasia. Fertil Steril 1994;61:401–402.

53. Gambrell RD Jr, Teran AZ: Changes in lipids and lipoproteins with long term estrogen deficiency and hormone replacement therapy. Am J Obstet Gynecol 1991;165:307–317.

54. Gapstur SM, Morrow M, Sellers TA: Hormone replacement and risk of breast cancer with a favorable histology: Results of the Iowa Women's Health Study. JAMA 1999; 281:2091–2097.

55. Gonnelli S, Cepollaro C, Pondrelli C et al: Ultrasound parameters in osteoporotic patients treated with salmon calcitonin: A longitudinal study. Osteoporosis Int 1996;6:303.

56. Goodman L, Awwad J, Marc K, et al: Continuous combined hormonal replacement therapy and the risk of endometrial cancer: Menopause. J N Am Menopause Soc 1994;1:57.

57. Grady B, Herrington D, Bittner V, et al: Cardiovascular disease outcomes during 6.8 years of hormone therapy (HERS II). JAMA 2002;288:49–57.

58. Greenblatt RB: The use of androgens in the menopause and other gynecic disorders. Obstet Gynecol Clin N Am 1987;14:251–268.

59. Greenlee RT, Hill-Harmon MB, Murray T, Thun M: Cancer statistics 2001. CA—Cancer J Clin 2001; 51:15–36.

60. Grodstein F, Stampher MJ, Colditz Ca, et al: Postmenopausal hormone therapy and mortality. New Engl J Med 1997;336:1769–1775.

61. Gruchow HW, Anderson AJ, Barborink JJ, et al: Postmenopausal use of estrogen and occlusion of coronary arteries. Am Heart J 1988;115:954.

62. Guerrieri JP, Elkas JC, Nash JD: Evaluating the endometrium in women on tamoxifen: a pilot study to compare a "gold standard" with and "old standard". Menopause: J N Am Menopause Soc 1997;4:6–9.

63. Gusberg SB: The individual at high risk for endometrial carcinoma. Am J Obstet Gynecol 1976;126:535.

64. Hammond CB, Jelovsek FR, Lee KL, et al: Effects of long-term estrogen replacement therapy: I-Metabolic. Am J Obstet Gynecol 1979;133:525.

65. Hammond CB, Jelovsek FR, Lee KL, et al: Effects of long-term estrogen replacement therapy: II-Neoplasia. Am J Obstet Gynecol 1979;133:537.

66. Hankinson SE, Colditz GA, Manson JE: A prospective study of birth control use and risk of breast cancer. Cancer Causes Control 1997; 8:65–72.

67. Hassis ST, Watts NB, Genant HK et al: Effects of risedronate treatment on vertebral and nonvertebral fractures in women with post menopausal osteoporosis. A randomized controlled trial. Vertebral efficacy with risedronate (VERT) study group. JAMA 1999: 282 (14) 1344–1352.

68. Henderson BE, Paganini-Hill A, Ross RK: Decreased mortality in users of estrogen replacement therapy. Arch Intern Med 1991;151:75–78.

69. Henderson S: Epidemiology of dementia. Ann Med Interns (Paris) 1998;149:181–186.

70. Hirsch AL, Stefanik ML, Stafford RS: National use of postmenopausal hormone therapy: annual trends and response to recent evidence. JAMA 2004;291:47–53.

71. Holmes MO, Hunter OH, Colditz GA: Association of dieting in dietary intake of patient and fatty acids with risk of breast cancer. JAMA 1999; 281:914–20.

72. Honjo H, Ogino Y, Naitoh K, et al: In vivo effects by estrone sulfate on the central nervous system: Senile dementia (Alzheimer's type). J Steroid Biochem 1989;34:521.

73. Honjo H, Tamura T, Matsumoto Y, et al: Estrogen as a growth factor to central nervous cells: Estrogen treatment promotes development of acetylcholinesterase: Positive forebrain neurons transplanted in anterior eye chamber. J Steroid Biochem Molec Biol 1992;41:633.

74. Honore LH: Increased incidence of symptomatic cholesterol cholelithiasis in perimenopausal women receiving estrogen replacement therapy. J Reprod Med 1980;25:187.

75. Hortobagyi GN, Hug V, Buzdar AU, et al: Sequential cyclic combined hormonal therapy for metastatic breast cancer. Cancer 1989;64:1002–1006.

76. Hulley S, Furberg C, Barrett-Connor E, et al, for the HERS Research Group: Cardiovascular disease outcomes during 6.8 years of hormone therapy: Heart and Estrogen/Progestin Replacement Study follow-up (HERS II). JAMA 2002; 288:58–66.

77. Hully S, Grady D, Bush T, et al: Randomized trial of estrogen plus progestin for secondary prevention of coronary heart disease in postmenopausal women (HERS). JAMA 1998;280:605–613.

78. Hunt K, Vessey M, McPherson K: Long-term surveillance of mortality and cancer incidence in women receiving hormone replacement therapy. Br J Obstet Gynaecol 1987;94:620–635.

79. Jamal A, Tivari RC, Murray T, Ward E, et al: Cancer Statistics, 2005, CA Cancer J Clin 2005; 55:10–30.

80. Jamal A, Thomas A, Murray T, Thum M: Cancer Statistics, 2002. CA Cancer J Clin 2002; 52: 23–47.

81. Kakar F, Weiss NS, Strite SA: Noncontraceptive estrogen use and the risk of gallstone disease in women. Am J Public Health 1988;78–564.

82. Kampen Dl, Sherwin BB: Estrogen use and verbal memory in healthy postmenopausal women. Obstet Gynecol 1994;83:979.

83. Karpf DH, Shapiro DR, Seeman E et al: Prevention of nonvertebral fractures by alendronate A metanalysis. Alendronate osteoporosis treatment study groups. JAMA 1997: 277(14) 1159–1164.

84. Katahn M, Pope J: The T-Factor, 2000 Diet. New York, WW Norton and Co., 1999.

85. Lauritzen C: Ostrogensubstitution in der postmenopause vor und nach behandeltem genital: Und mammakarzinom. Menopause Hormone substitution Heute 1993;6:76–88.

86. Lauritzen C, Meier F: Risks of endometrial and mammary cancer morbidity and mortality in long-term estrogen treatment. In: The Climacteric: An Update. Van Herendael H & B, et al (eds.) Lancaster, England: MTP Press, Ltd., 1984;207–216.

87. Leather AT, Savvas M, Studd JWW: Endometrial histology and bleeding patterns after 8 years of continuous combined estrogen and progestogen therapy. Obstet Gynecol 1991; 78:1008.

88. Levgur M: Hormone therapy for women after breast cancer: a review. J Reprod Med 2004;49:510–526.

89. Li CI, Weiss NS, Stanford JL, Daling JR: Hormone replacement therapy in relation to risk of lobular and ductal breast carcinoma in middle-aged women. Cancer 2000; 88:2570–2577.

90. Lind T, Cameron FC, Hunter FM, et al: A prospective controlled trial of six forms of hormone replacement therapy given to postmenopausal women. Br J Obstet Gynaecol 1979;86:1.

91. Looker AC, Orwoll ES, Johnston CC Jr, et al: Prevelance of low femoral bone density in older U.S. adults. From N Hanes III, J Bone Mineral Res. 1997: 12: 1769–1771.

92. MacDougall DS. Meeting highlights: Third international symposium on osteoporosis.Drug Ther 1991; 21:40.

93. Mack TM, Pike MC, Henderson BE, et al: Estrogens and endometrial cancer in a retirement community. N Engl J Med 1976;294:1262.

94. Magnusson C, Baron JA, Correia N, Berger GS, Dami HO, Persson I: Breast cancer risk following long-term oestrogen and oestrogen-progestin replacement therapy. Int J Cancer 1999; 81:339–44.

95. Maki PM: WHIMS findings: Do they apply to women who begin HT around menopause. Council on Hormone Education. Montvale, NJ, Advanstar Medical Economics 2004; 2:3–8.

96. Maki PM, Resnick SM: Longitudinal effects of estrogen replacement therapy on PET cerebral blood flow and cognition. Neurobiol Aging 2000; 21:373–383.

97. Mann JI, Vessey MP, Thorogood M, et al: Myocardial infarction in young women with special reference to oral contraceptive practice. Br Med J 1975;2:241.

98. Mauvais-Jarvis P, Sitruk-Ware R, Kuttem F: Luteal phase defect and breast cancer genesis. Breast Cancer Res Treat 1982;2:139.

99. McClung MR, Guesens P, Miller PD et al: Effect of risedronate on the risk of hip fracture in elderly women. Hip intervention program study group. N Engl J Med 2001;344:333–340.

100. McFarland KF, Boniface ME, Boniface ME, Hornung CA, et al: Risk factors and noncontraceptive estrogen use in women with and without coronary disease. Am Heart J 1989; 117:1209.

101. McMichael AJ, Potter JD: Host factors in carcinogenesis. Certain bile-acid metabolic profiles that selectively increase the risk of proximal colon cancer. J Natl Cancer Inst 1985;75:185.

102. Nabulsi A, Folsom AR, White A, et al: Association of hormone-replacement therapy with various cardiovascular risk factors in postmenopausal women. N Engl J Med 1993;328:1609.

103. Nachtigall LE, Nachtigall RH, Nachtigall RB, et al: Estrogen replacement II: A prospective study in the relationship to carcinoma and cardiovascular and metabolic problems. Obstet Gynecol 1979;54:74.

104. Nachtigall MJ, Smilen SW, Nachtigall RD, et al: Incidence of breast cancer in a 22-year study of women receiving estrogen-progestin replacement therapy. Obstet Gynecol 1992;80:827–830.

105. National Cancer Institute: Surveillance, Epidemiology and End Results (SEER). Bethesda, Biometry Branch of the National Cancer Institute, 1980, p 47.

106. Natrajan PK, Soumakis K, Gamrbell RD Jr: Estrogen replacement therapy in women with previous breast cancer. Am J Obstet Gynecol 1999;181:228–95.

107. Natrajan PK, Gambrell RD Jr: Estrogen replacement therapy in patients with early breast cancer. Am J Obstet Gynecol 2002;187:289–295.

108. Neer RM, Arnaud CD, Zanchetta Jr et al: Effect of parathyroid hormone (1–34) on fractures and bone mineral density in postmenopausal women with osteoporosis. N Engl J Med 2001:344; 1434–1441.

109. Newcombe PA, Storer BE: Postmenopausal hormone use and risk of large-bowel cancer. J Natl Cancer Inst 1995;87:1067.

110. Notelovitz M: Exercise, nutrition, and the coagulation effects of estrogen replacement on cardiovascular health. Obstet Gynecol Clin N Am 1987;14:121–141.

111. O'Meara ES, Rossing MA, Darling Jr, et al: Hormone replacement therapy after a diagnosis of breast cancer in relation to recurrence and mortality. J Natl Cancer Inst 2001;93:754–762.

112. Padwick MC, Pryse-Davies J, Whitehead MI: A simple method determining the optimal dosage of progestin in postmenopausal women receiving estrogens. N Enlg J Med 1986;315:930.

113. Paganini-Hill A, Henderson VW: Estrogen deficiency and risk of Alzheimer's disease in women. Am J Epidemiol 1994;140:256.

114. Paganini-Hill A, Ross RK, Henderson BE: Postmenopausal oestrogen treatment and stroke: A prospective study. Br Med J 1988;297:519.

115. Peck WA, Barrett-Conner E, Buckwalter JA, Gambrell RD Jr, et al: Consensus conference: Osteoporosis. JAMA 1984;252:799.

116. Pentitti DB, Perlman JA, Sidney S: Noncontraceptive estrogens and mortality: Long-term follow-up of women in the Walnut Creek study. Obstet Gynecol 1987;70:289.

117. Perez-Jaraiz MD, Revilla M, Alvarez de los Heros JI et al: Proplylaxis of osteoporosis with calcium, estrogens, and/or eelcatonin: Comparative longitudinal study of bone mass. Maturitas 1996;23:327.

118. Persson I, Yuen J, Bergkvist L, et al: (Letter) Combined estrogen-progestogen replacement and breast cancer risk. Lancet 1992;340:1044.

119. Petranik K, Kable WT, Bewtra C, Gallager JC: (Abstract) Use of progestin challenge test in elderly women: Menopause. J N Am Menopause Soc 1995;2:278.

120. Plu-Bureau G, Le MG Sitruk-Ware R, et al: Progestogen use and decreased risk of breast cancer in a cohort study of premenopausal women with benign breast disease. Br J Cancer 1994; 70:270–277.

121. Powles TH, Opfell RW, Margileth DA: Hormone replacement therapy after bresat cancer. Lancet 1993; 342:60–61.

122. Prior JC: Progesterone as a bone-trophic hormone. Endocrin Rev 1990;11:368.

123. Punnonen R, Lammintansta R, Erkkda R, et al: Estradiol valerate therapy and the renin-aldosterone system in castrated women. Maturitas 1980;2:91.

124. Ray NF, Chan JK, Thamer et al: Medical expenditures for the treatment of osteoporotic fractures in 1995: report from National Ostetoporosis Foundation J Bone Mineral Res. 1997;12:24–35.

125. Riggs BL, Melton LJ III: The world wide problem of osteroporsis: Insight afforded by epidemiology. Bone 1995: 17 (Suppl.5) 505–511.

126. Ron E, Lunenfeld B, Menczer J, et al: Cancer incidence in a cohort of infertile women. Am J Epidemiol 1987; 125:780–790.

127. Rosen C, Mallinak N, Cain D et al: A comparison of biochemical markers in monitoring skeletal responses to hormone replacement therapy in early postmenopausal women. Bone Miner Res 1996;11:5119.

128. Rosner B, Colditz GA. Nurses Health Study: Coincidence mathematical model of breast cancer incidence. J Natl Cancer Inst 1996; 88:359–64.

129. Ross P.D: Clinical consequences of vertebral fractures. Amer J Med 1997: 103:30–42 (S).

130. Ross RK, Paganini-Hill A, Wan PC, et al: Effect of hormone replacement therapy on breast cancer risk: Estrogen versus estrogen plus progestin. J Natl Cancer Inst 2000; 92:328–332.

131. Rossouw JE, Anderson GL, Prentice RI, et al: Risks and benefits of estrogen plus progestin in healthy postmenopausal women: principal results from the Women's Health Initiative randomized controlled trial. JAMA 2002;288:321–333.

132. Sarles H, Gerolami A, Cros RC: Diet and cholesterol gallstones: A further study. Digestion 1978;17:128.

133. Sarrel PM: Blood flow. In: Treatment of the Postmenopausal Woman: Basic and Clinical Aspects, RA Lobo, (ed.). New York, Raven Press, 1994, pp 251–262.

134. Sarrel PM: Sexuality in the middle years. Obstet Gynecol Clin N Am 1987;15:49–62.

135. Sattin RW, Rulin GL, Webster LA et al: Family history and risk of breast cancer. JAMA 1985; 253:1908.

136. Schairer L, Gail M, Byrne C, et al: Estrogen replacement therapy and breast cancer survival in a large screening study. J Nat Cancer Inst 1999; 91:264–270.

137. Schairer L, Lubin J, Troisi R, Sturgeon S, Brinton L, Hoover R: Menopause estrogen and estrogen-progestin replacement therapy and breast cancer risk. JAMA 2000; 283: 485–91.

138. Schlesselman JJ Net effect of oral contraceptive use on the risk of cancer of women in the United States. Obstet Gynecol 1995;85:793.

139. Schumaker SA, Legaut C, Thai SL et al: Estrogen plus progestin and the incidence of dementia and mild cognitive impairment in postmenopausal women. JAMA 2003, 289:2651–2662.

140. Schumaker SA, Legault C, Kuller L, et al: Conjugated equine estrogens and incidence of probable dementia and mild cognitive impairment in postmenopausal women, JAMA 2004; 291:2947–2958.

141. Shapiro S, Kelly JP, Rosenberg L, et al: Risk of localized and widespread endometrial cancer in relation to recent and discontinued use of conjugated estrogens. N Engl J Med 1985;313:969.

142. Sherwin BB, Gelfand MM: Differential symptom response to parenteral estrogen and/or androgen administration in the surgical menopause. Am J Obstet Gynecol 1985;151:153.

143. Sillero-Arenas M, Delgado-Rodriguez M, Rodigues-Canteras R, et al: Menopausal hormone replacement therapy and breast cancer: A meta-analysis. Obstet Gynecol 1972;79:286.

144. Smith DC, Prentice R, Thompson DJ, et al: Association of exogenous estrogen and endometrial carcinoma. N Engl J Med 1975;293:1164.

145. Speroff L: A clinician demurs. Sexuality, Reproduction, and Menopause 2003; 1:15–18.

146. Stampfer MJ, Grodstein F: Role of hormone replacement in cardiovascular disease. In: Treatment of the Postmenopausal Woman: Basic and Clinical Aspects, RA Lobo, (ed.). New York, Raven Press, 1994, pp 223–233.

147. Stampfer MJ, Willet WC, Colditz GA, et al: A Prospective study of postmenopausal estrogen therapy and coronary heart disease. N Engl J Med 1985;313:1044.

148. Stanczyk FZ, Shoupe D, Nunez V, et al: A randomized comparison of non-oral estradiol delivery in postmenopausal women. Am J Obstet Gynecol 1988;159:1540.

149. Stanford JL, Weiss NS, Voight LF et al: Combined estrogen and progestin hormone replacement therapy in relation to risk of breast cancer in middle-aged women. JAMA 1995;274:137–142.

150. Stoll BA, Parbhoo S: Treatment of menopausal symptoms in breast cancer patients. Lancet 1988;1:1278–1279.

151. Strickland DM, Gambrell RD Jr, Butzin CA, et al: The relationship between breast cancer survival and prior postmenopausal estrogen use. Obstet Gynecol 1992;80:400–404.

152. Strickler RC: Women's Health Initiative Results: A glass more empty than full. Fertil Steril 2003;80:488–490.

153. Studd J, Magos A: Hormone pellet implantation for the menopause and premenstrual syndrome. Obstet Gynecol Clin N Am 1987;14:229–249.

154. Studd JWW: The climacteric syndrome. In: Female and Male Climacteric. Serr DM, van Keep PA, Greenblatt RB (eds.) Lancaster, England: MTP Press, Ltd., 1979, p 23.

155. Sulak PJ, Crubel P, Lane R: Efficacy and safety of a constant-estrogen, pulsed progestin regimen in hormone replacement therapy. Int J Fertil 1999;44: 286–296.

156. Sullivan JM, Zwagg RV, Lemp GF, et al: Postmenopausal estrogen use and coronary atherosclerosis. Ann Intern Med 1988;108:358.

157. Tang M-X, Jacobs D, Stern Y et al: Effect of oestrogen during menopause on risk and age at onset of Alzheimer's disease. Lancet 1996;348:429.

158. The Coronary Drug Project Research Group: The coronary drug project: Initial findings leading to modifications of its research protocol. JAMA 1970; 214: 1303.

159. The Women's Health Initiative Steering Committee: Effect of conjugated equine estrogens in postmenopausal women with hysterectomy. The Women's Health Initiative randomized controlled trial. JAMA 2004;291:1701–1712.

160. Thom MH, White PJ, Williams RM, et al: Prevention and treatment of endometrial disease in climacteric women receiving oestrogen therapy. Lancet 1979; 2:455.

161. Thomas HV, Key TJ, Allen DS: Reversal of relation between BMI and endogenous estrogens concentration with menopausal status, J. Natl Cancer Inst 1997; 89: 396–398.

162. Tonino RP, Merimier PJ, Emkey R et al: Skelltal benefits of alendronate: 7 year treatment of post menopausal osteoporotic women. Phase III Osteoporosis treatment study group. J Clin Endocrinol Metal 2000: 85(9) 3109–3115.

163. Toran-Allerand CD: Estrogen as a treatment for Alzheimer's disease. (Letter) JAMA 2000;284:307–308.

164. Torgerson DJ, Bell Syer SE: Hormone replacement and prevention of non vertebral fractures - a metanaylsis of randomized trials. JAMA 2001: 285: 2891–2897.

165. Uric-Vrscaj M, Bebar S: A case control study of hormone replacement therapy after primary surgical breast cancer treatment. Eur J Surg Oncol 1999;25: 146–151.

166. Ursin G, Henderson BE, Haile RW: Does birth control use increase the risk of breast cancer in women with BRCA1/BRCA2, mutation more than in other women? Cancer Res 1997; 57: 3678–3681.

167. Vassilopoulou-Selin R, Asmar L, Hortobagi GN, et al: Estrogen replacement therapy after localized breast cancer. Clinical outcome of 319 women followed prospectively. J. Clin Oncol 1999; 17:1482–1487.

168. Virsin G, Ross RR, Sullivan J, Hamisch R, Henderson B, Bernstein L: Use of birth control and risk of breast cancer in young women. Breast Cancer Res Treat 1998; 80:175–84.

169. Voherr H: Oral contraceptives and hormone replacement therapy: Are progestogens and progestins breast mitogens? Am J Obstet Gynecol 1986;155:1140–1142.

170. Wentz WB: Progestin therapy in endometrial hyperplasia. Gynecol Oncol 1974;2:362.

171. Wile AG, Opfell RW, Marileth DA: Hormone replacement therapy in previously treated breast cancer patients. Am J Surg 1993;165:372–375.

172. Willis DB, Calle EE, Miracle-McMahill HL, et al: Estrogen replacement therapy and ris of fatal breast cancer in a prospective cohort of postmenopausal women in the United States. Cancer Causes and Control 1996;7:449–457.

173. Wilson PW, Garrison RJ, Willet WC, et al: Postmenopausal estrogen use, cigarette smoking, and cardiovascular morbidity in women over 50: The Framingham Study. N Engl J Med 1985;313:1038.

174. Wingo PA, Lee NC, Ory HW et al: Age-specific differences in the relationship between oral contraceptive use and breast cancer. Obstet Gynecol 1991;78:161.

175. Wren BO, Routledge AD: The effect of type and dose of oestrogen on the blood pressure of postmenopausal women. Maturitas 1983;5:135.

176. Yager JO, Liehr JG: Molecular mechanism oestrogen carcinogenesis. Ann Rev Pharmacol Toxicol 1996; 36: 203–32.

177. Zandi PP, Carlson MC, Plassman BL, et al: Hormone replacement therapy and incidence of Alzheimer's disease in older women. The Cache County study. JAMA 2002;288:2123–2129.

178. Ziel HK, Finkle WD: Increased risk of endometrial carcinoma among users of conjugated estrogens. N Engl J Med 1975;293:1167.

MANUFACTURER'S LIST

Barr Laboratories, Inc.
400 Chestnut Ridge Road
Woodcliff Lake, NJ 07677
800 222 0190

Berlex Laboratories
300 Fairfield road
Wayne, NJ 07470
973 694 4100

Duramed Pharmaceuticals, Inc.
5040 Lester Road
Cincinnati, OH 45214
800 222 0190

King Pharmaceuticals, Inc.
501 Fifth Street
Bristol, TN 37620
800 776 3637

Novartis Pharmaceutical Corporation
One Health Plaza
East Hanover, NJ 07936-1080
862 778 8300

Ortho-McNeil Pharmaceuticals
1000 U. S. Route 202 South
Raritan, NJ 08869
800 682 6532

Pharmacia, Inc.
7000 Post Road
Dublin, OH 43016

Solvay Pharmaceuticals
901 Sawyer Road
Marietta, GA 30062
770 578 9000

Warner Chilcott Laboratories
Rockaway 80 Corporate Center
100 Enterprise Drive, Suite 280
Rockaway, NJ 07866
800 521 8813

Wyeth-Ayerst Pharmaceuticals
Division of American Home Products Corporation
P O Box 8299
Philadelphia, PA 19101
800 934 5556

Invitation from EMIS, Inc.

You are invited to visit our web site to order additional center-indexed books, or share comments.

www.emispub.com

REPRODUCTIVE HEALTH

Breastfeeding: A Problem Solving Manual
by Carroll, Johnson & Saunders
ISBN 0-929240-68-5

Contraceptive Surgery for Men and Women 2nd ed.
by William M. Moss/AVSC
ISBN 0-929240-26-X

Gynecological Care Manual for HIV Positive Women
by Risa Denenberg, FNP
ISBN 0-929240-58-8

Managing Contraceptive Pill Patients—12th ed.
by Richard P. Dickey, MD, PhD
ISBN 0-917634-31-4

Mid-Life Sexuality: Enrichment and Problem Solving
by James P. Semmens, MD
ISBN 0-929240-20-0

CARDIOLOGY

Cholesterol Treatment: A Guide to Lipid Disorder Management
by David A. Leaf, MD
ISBN 0-917634-02-0

Emergency Cardiac Maneuvers 2nd ed.
by Carl E. Bartechhi, MD
ISBN 0-929240-15-4

Management of Heart Failure
by Jay N. Cohen, MD & Spencer H. Kubo, MD
ISBN 0-929240-17-0

Management of Hypertension—8th ed.
by Norman M. Kaplan, MD
ISBN 0-917634-10-1

GENERAL MEDICINE

A Manual on Drug Dependence
by Gabriel G. Nahas, MD, PhD
ISBN 0-929240-46-4

A Practical Anesthesia Information Guide
by Raymond J. Jerome, MD
ISBN 0-929240-21-9

Arthritis Therapy: A Clinician's Manual
by Thomas G. Kantor, MD
ISBN 0-929240-40-5

Breast Disease in Women and Men: Handbook
by Pamela A Shuler, D.NSc.
ISBN 0-929240-54-5

CEO Guide to Health Facility Development 2nd ed.
Hershel E. Weeks, PhD
ISBN 0-929240-47-2

Handbook of Headache Disorders, 2nd ed.
Arthur Elkind, MD
ISBN 0-929240-62-6

Management of Aneurysmal Subaracnoid Hemorrhage
by Damirez Fossett, MD
ISBN 0-929240-59-6

Medical Management of Depression—3rd ed.
by Charles DeBattista, DMH, MD & Ira D. Glick, MD
ISBN 0-917634-09-8

Oxidative Balance: Antioxidant Lifestyle
by David A. Leaf, MD & Peter Glassman, PhD
ISBN 0-917634-01-2

Projective Psychodiagnostic Assessment
by H. Stephen Caldwell, PhD & Stacey L. Dixon, PhD
ISBN 0-929240-49-9

Readers are invited to send suggestions for changes and new information they believe should be included in *Hormone Replacement Therapy, Sixth Edition,* to the author, in care of the publisher at our web site: www.emispub.com., click on *Ask the Author*. If the information is used, the sender will receive a complimentary copy of the next printing of *Hormone Replacement Therapy*. New information is often added to each printing.